I'VE FALLEN

AND

I <u>CAN</u>

GET UP!

I'VE FALLEN

AND

I CAN

GET UP!

*The Ultimate Life
Recovery Program*

DR. CHRISTOPHER R. MILLER

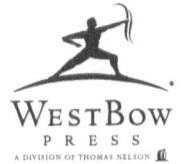

WESTBOW
PRESS
A DIVISION OF THOMAS NELSON

WestBow Press books may be ordered through booksellers or by contacting:

WestBow Press
A Division of Thomas Nelson
1663 Liberty Drive
Bloomington, IN 47403
www.westbowpress.com
1-(866) 928-1240

ISBN: 978-1-4497-1580-9 (sc)
ISBN: 978-1-4497-1581-6 (hc)
ISBN: 978-1-4497-1579-3 (e)

Library of Congress Control Number: 2011927020

Printed in the United States of America

WestBow Press rev. date: 05/02/2011

AUTHOR'S NOTE

Every effort has been made to ensure that the contents of this book are accurate. The author is not engaged in rendering professional advice or services to the individual reader. The ideas and strategies in this book are not intended as a substitute for consulting your physician. All matters regarding your health require medical supervision. The author shall not be liable for any loss or damage arising from the views expressed herein.

Portions of this book can be used as a self-treatment for more mild forms of depression and anxiety—those individuals not requiring the services of a psychiatrist or psychologist—but who are merely in need of a mental tune-up. Or, it can be used as a supplement to therapy sessions for individuals who are in treatment.

Of course, there are times when professional treatment is most certainly warranted. You should consider consulting a mental health professional if:

you feel hopeless or suicidal;

you have been depressed for at least four weeks and have not improved in spite of your own best efforts;

you have strong sexual or violent impulses you cannot control;

you hear voices or have hallucinations or experience unusual occurrences that others cannot seem to understand;

you are abusing drugs or alcohol;

you find yourself further isolating from others;

you feel overwhelmed and discouraged and cannot seem to function at work or in school.

All client identities, as well as specifics regarding their cases, have been altered to protect privacy.

To my children, Christopher and Madison:

May this book serve as a comfort and guide through times of difficulty. May you always strive to realize all that God has set before you, both for time, and for eternity.

and

To my brother, Richard R. Miller III ("Rich"):

Against incredible odds, and having courageously passed through treacherous terrain, you got back up. I have tremendous respect and admiration for you!

and

To Mom:

In loving appreciation for your unfailing support since day one, and for serving as a model of unconditional love.

Failure is only the opportunity to more intelligently begin again.

-Henry Ford

TABLE OF CONTENTS

PREFACE

The Get Up! formula for success is rooted in both physical and social science evidence-based research and the experience of thousands of men and women over the centuries who have applied similar principles and techniques with outstanding results. Therefore, as you read, become inspired, and apply this amazing formula, you can do so with absolute confidence.

The Central Goal of Get Up!

The central goal of Get Up! is to help individuals who are struggling with failure, burnout, discouragement, hopelessness, despair, or even the depressing malaise of mediocrity learn that a bright future is indeed possible, and to immediately begin the journey towards what I like to call *ultimate life recovery.*

Years of research and clinical practice have proven that life transformation, i.e., ultimate life recovery, is best accomplished via the realm of the brain and its accompanying thoughts—commonly identified as *cognition* (cognition refers to the psychological structures, processes, and thoughts that shape our perspectives about, and reactions to, life events).

What is the reason that ultimate life recovery can best be accomplished via the realm of the brain and its accompanying thoughts?

Because your thoughts are incredibly powerful! So powerful in fact, that in the ancient scriptures the book of Genesis (chapter 11 and verse 6) records that God sought to confuse the language of the ancient

Babylonians for having set out to build a tower to heaven, stating as a reason, "[because] nothing they intend [have in mind] to do shall be impossible to them."

God confused the language of the Babylonians because although their thoughts were indeed powerful, they appeared to be trusting in themselves without reference to God's design and purposes for humanity.

The power of the mind, and a person's will and intentions, are always best utilized in keeping with God's divine law of love, and not for selfishly ambitious ends. Otherwise, our efforts eventually come to have very little meaning, as this story so richly illustrates.

Thoughts carry with them the power to build or tear down, to motivate or depress, to breed life or promote death. That is why in matters related to personal transformation (or "life overhaul" if you will), a healthy brain and thought life deserve our undivided attention as a first order priority.

The Engine in You

Ask yourself this question, "If I paid an auto mechanic to give my fifteen year old, 250,000 mile car a major overhaul and he or she completed the job without even so much as touching the engine, would I be satisfied?" The obvious answer is a resounding "No!"

You would probably protest the bill, arguing, "You didn't even touch the engine! Why should I pay?" And you would be right.

Regardless of how well the shocks, struts, brakes, wheels, tires, and electrical sensors are working, if the engine is not functioning properly, you are not likely to get very far down the road!

This analogy parallels the relationship between your brain (the engine) and your ability to live successfully (the objective of the overhaul).

For that reason, the formula and strategies described in this book are essentially *brain* and *thought* based.

Expressing You

Just as the engine of your car is central to a multitude of vital components and systems necessary for proper function, so your brain and its thoughts are central to virtually every aspect of your life, e.g., maintaining strong and nurturing relationships, making healthy life choices, clear communication, focused attention, and ultimately, your soulful connections—love and spiritual growth.

According to clinical neuroscientist and psychiatrist Dr. Daniel Amen (2002),

We can now see actual evidence of this brain-soul connection through the latest brain-imaging techniques . . . These studies have so clearly taught me that when the brain is healthy we are compassionate, thoughtful, loving, relaxed, and goal-directed, and when the brain is sick or damaged we are unfeeling, impulsive, angry, tense, and unfocused, and it is very hard for our souls and our relationship with God to be at peace . . . a dynamic feedback loop exists between the brain and the events of our lives [parenting, social interactions, vocation, etc.]. The brain impacts our behavior, and how we behave impacts actual brain function. Our latest research has shown that thoughts, feelings, and social interactions all impact brain function in potentially positive and negative ways . . . it is likely that Mother Teresa and Mahatma Gandhi had optimal brain function . . . it is also likely that Adolf Hitler and other brutal dictators had faulty brain wiring, despite being able to rise to power . . . new research . . . suggests that the brain influences and may, in fact, be wired to experience God or deep spirituality.

Amazingly, without the advantages of modern research, William Shakespeare poetically, powerfully, and quite prophetically referred to the brain as "the soul's fragile dwelling place."

If we recognize the brain does all the things that we (traditionally) attributed to the soul, then God must have some way of interacting with human brains.

-Nancy Murphy, Philosopher of Science and Religion at the Fuller Seminary, Pasadena

Towards a Cognitive Approach

Over the years, mental health research has consistently recognized the effectiveness of cognitive forms of therapy in dealing with a variety of clinical issues. Depression, general anxiety, obsessive compulsive disorder (OCD), and post-traumatic stress disorder (PTSD) represent just a sample of the clinical issues for which cognitive based approaches to therapy are deemed particularly effective.

Researchers and practitioners in the fields of neuroscience, education, psychotherapy, hypnotherapy, and life coaching are becoming increasingly aware of both the power and potential of cognition, and of the brain's ability to respond constructively to interventions that are applied well.

What Scientists are Saying

Over the past decade and a half, fascinating breakthroughs in neuroscience (in large part due to advanced brain imaging technology which has improved tremendously since its initial introduction to medicine roughly three decades ago) has shifted the scientific community towards a common acceptance (and celebration!) of brain *plasticity* (brain plasticity is a term often used by neuroscientists in describing the brain's ability to change, modify, reprogram, and reorganize).

Mary ET Boyle, Ph.D. and cognitive scientist at the University of California, San Diego (UCSD) suggests that neuroplasticity and brain reorganization represents the direction of neuroscience as we know it today (Boyle, 2010). Dr. Boyle's teachings coincide with the perspectives of many, and quite probably most, neuroscientists.

Not long ago, the prevailing view was that the brain remained "fixed" or "crystallized" throughout a person's life. Author and scientist Eric Jensen contends that while we have always known that the ". . . brain was smaller in childhood; once it reached maturity, we thought it remained more or less stable over many years before beginning to deteriorate somewhat with age. This view of a 'static' brain is decidedly out of date. Yes, the most amazing new discovery about the brain might be that *human beings have the capacity and the choice to be able to change our own brains"* (Jensen, 2005).

Cacioppo, Berntson, Sheridan, and McClintock (2001) provide evidence that environmental events at one level of an organism (molecules, cells, organs, and individual behavior) can profoundly affect events at other levels. This research finding suggests that your choices, experiences, and actions can actually lead to changes in your brain.

Additionally, researchers have reportedly discovered evidence of social influence with regard to both the constitution (the substance) of genes (Reik, Dean, & Walter, 2001), and their expressive function (Suomi, 1999). The implication being that environmental triggers, such as stress (Foster & Cairns, 1994), can radically alter our genes through reprogramming, so that we can in fact influence our genetic material.

According to Jensen (2005), "The result of the various interrelation of humans shaping environments and environments shaping humans is that there is no fixed human brain; it is always a work in progress. . . . Your brain is dynamic and constantly changing as a result of the world you live in and life you lead. . . . Your brain is a cauldron of changing chemicals, electrical activity, cell growth, cell death, connectivity, and change."

In the fine wording of the physiologist, psychologist, and philosopher William James (1890),

Plasticity . . . means the possession of a structure weak enough to yield to an influence, but strong enough not to yield all at once. Each relatively stable phase of equilibrium in such a structure is marked by what we may call a new set of habits. Organic matter, especially nervous tissue, seems endowed with a very extraordinary degree of plasticity of this sort; so that we may without hesitation lay down . . . that the phenomena of habit in living beings are due to the plasticity of the organic materials of which their bodies are composed.

The ability to influence genetic structures is a powerful revelation. It removes the daunting belief that we are somehow born with genetic limitations that cannot be overcome.

Echoes of the Motivational Classics

These studies and many more like them echo what authors of self-help literature have been writing for decades, namely, that a person's brain (and hence, his or her life) is not fixed, i.e., an individual is not a victim of his or her perceived limitation, be it genetic or environmental. But rather, the brain can be changed, modified, and reprogrammed to support whatever is in a person's heart of hearts to become, regardless of circumstance.

What Napoleon Hill in his classic work *Think and Grow Rich* pioneered (through qualitative research, having interviewed many of the world's wealthiest individuals in hopes of discovering their secrets to success) and eloquently expressed in awe-inspiring language, powerfully attests to the very discoveries only recently verified by the scientific community. He and others like him knew both intuitively, as well as from personal experience, what research so many decades later confirmed: "Whatever the mind can conceive and believe, the mind can achieve" (Hill, 1937).

If you sincerely desire to make significant changes in your life, you can. Your part is to want (i.e., *desire* and *intentionality*) change *and* be willing to apply the principles (e.g., *courage, discipline,* and *persistence*) outlined in this book to your life.

One Little Step

If the prospect of starting over and rebuilding your life seems like a daunting task, than perhaps you will find encouragement from a Chinese proverb, which says, "even the longest trip starts with one little step."

Introducing New Mind Synergy

After a decade and a half of private practice, research, and plenty of personal experiences of falling flat on my face!, I have developed a coaching formula that produces tremendous results for people in search of solutions to many of the common stumbling blocks that contribute to failure in their lives. I call it New Mind Synergy.

New Mind Synergy maximizes cognition and goals, the two most powerful elements necessary for change, and combines them into one dynamic coaching formula, New Mind Synergy = Cognition and Goals Squared (NMS=CG2). The net result of applying this formula is the following: a synergistic explosion of awakened possibility, newfound freedom, and personal power—*dunamis*—a Greek term from which we derive the word "dynamite."

The word "synergy" also happens to come from an ancient Greek term, *syn-ergos,* which is used to describe the compounding phenomenon of two or more agents working together, achieving considerably more than two agents acting independently could achieve, and resulting in an end product that is greater than the sum of its parts.

How New Mind Synergy Works

New Mind Synergy seeks to optimize cognition as expressed by a healthy, balanced, productive thought life in conjunction with the power of goals. So I have divided the book into two parts accordingly.

I am often asked, "Which is more important, cognition or goals?" What is the answer? "Both!" A healthy mind set allows you to realize your goals more clearly, while a passion filled personal goals blueprint fuels some amazing positive cognitive energy, resulting in a dynamic explosion of personal power and increased self confidence.

How New Mind Synergy Changed My Life

When I discovered the dynamic effects of combining proper mind care with the power of goals, both my personal life and my private practice shifted significantly in a very positive direction.

As I tapped into who I really am at the core, and what I truly want for my life, I became enthusiastically infused with the power to begin the journey of realizing all that is in my heart of hearts to achieve.

Not that I became somebody altogether different but that I woke up to who I really am and what I truly desire deep inside. For me, it took a life crisis to finally reach that point. As you read the body of the book, you will quickly see why I have such an optimistic attitude about life crises', because they serve as a wake-up call, alerting us to the necessity of, and new opportunities for, renewal.

I suddenly found myself launched on an exciting adventure full of possibility. I became more confident, focused, and disciplined.

No longer did I have to wander around the mountain of confusion, hopelessness, and despair. I began to finally see my life and its purpose more clearly. My deepest inner passions were now being realized and expressed in a powerful, new, fun (yes fun!), and dynamic way.

This discovery was exciting for me then, and the excitement increases with each passing day.

My clients have benefitted by this new love affair with possibility, and my interventions more hopeful and focused than ever, seem to have a very positive effect on their progress as well.

The Good News

The good news is that anyone, anywhere, at any time, can apply this same, easy to use, New Mind Synergy formula for success. Whether you feel hopeless, confused, and discouraged, or are merely in need of a tune-up, New Mind Synergy produces potentially life transforming results.

I have confidence that if you apply these principles, you will do exceptionally well. I am rooting for you!

-The Author

INTRODUCTION

Beginning over, *again*? Have you fallen down and want to get back up, but aren't quite sure how? Perfect. That's a good place to be—a little bit humbled and hungry for change!

The truth is, whether you are a stay-at-home parent, corporate CEO, doctor, lawyer, Indian chief, "butcher, baker, or candlestick maker," and regardless of how many zero's are stacked behind your bank account digits, not one person on this planet is immune from loneliness, failure, set-backs, personal defeat, or even the depressing malaise of mediocrity.

Maybe you're struggling with a significant loss? It could be the devastating loss of a loved one—through death, an estranged child, or a broken marriage—your home, your way of life, or a career or business failure.

Maybe you are struggling with depression—a symptom of the chasm between your life presently and where your heart of hearts longs to be. Or perhaps you find yourself repeating patterns of self-defeating behavior, such as, continuing in unhealthy relationships, or practicing an addiction that threatens to destroy you?

Possibly it is an overwhelming combination of things that makes starting over seem virtually impossible? You feel overwhelmed, discouraged, or even hopeless.

Roadmap to Ultra-recovery

This book, laid out in an intimate fifteen session coaching format, reinforced with fascinating and heartwarming experiences of real life clients, serves as your road map to what I call *ultra-recovery*. *Ultra*-because you don't want to just recover what you had before—you want to ultra-recover, i.e., discover a far greater way of life than would have been possible had the unfortunate event(s) not occurred.

There is Hope for You

You may be thinking, "You don't know my story. I just think I'm too far gone, and there is no hope left for me!" Well if that is you, then I invite you to read further. You see, I believe that there is always hope for every person who desires a new direction in life. In fact, the depths of despair you may be feeling could very well represent an emerging turning point in your life.

It is when we feel beaten down by life and our wounds are raw and throbbing with pain that our awareness is quickened. We see clearly that a problem exists, and we become motivated to search for solutions. As Albert Einstein once said, "The problems you face cannot be solved at the same level of awareness that created them."

Let Your Journey Begin

Could this dark night of the soul serve as a curious beckoning, calling you to explore untapped reservoirs of possibility that have lay dormant within you all along?

Could this book offer clues that will assist you in discovering many of the answers to your life's disappointments, launching you on a journey of personal success and fulfillment beyond anything you could have ever imagined? The answer is a resounding "Yes!"

Your Springboard to Success Has Arrived

As a result of our time together, the personal insights you will learn can virtually launch you towards a richer, more meaningful and successful life—the life you've dreamed of for years, but always seemed to fall short of obtaining. The fear, confusion, doubt, and insecurity that mark your present reality will fade like darkness before the rising sun. Confidently, you will burst forth into a new life of clarity, renewed strength, and inspired purpose.

The Get Up! New Mind Synergy success formula forms the basis for this book, and contains a compilation of the very best of more than fifteen years of personal experience, human study, counseling, and coaching practice. As you read, you will discover what I and countless others have discovered: there is no problem so great, no situation so hopeless, no habit so deeply rooted, that it cannot be overcome.

Change is Possible

By linking powerful mind-transforming techniques (cognitive interventions, Part One) with your deepest inner passions (expressed through goals, Part Two), a New Mind Synergy is created (repeated here for those who skipped through the Preface) and expressed as follows: "synergy" originates from the ancient Greek term *syn-ergos,* which is used to describe the compounding phenomena of two or more agents working together, achieving considerably more than two single agents acting independently could achieve, and resulting in an end product that is greater than the sum of its parts. This results in a new, more powerful thought life—a new, more powerful *you*!

What to Expect

In Part One (Sessions One through Two), Get Up! unflinchingly sheds light on many of the most common reasons we fail. Sometimes our wounds are self-inflicted—aren't you tired of going round-and-round the mountain of repeated self-defeating thoughts and behaviors? Also, we will review some contributors to failure that lie outside of our control, i.e., external factors. Get Up! then introduces a variety of insightful and practical remedies to assist in your journey towards personal freedom (Sessions Three through Six).

An "aha" moment (where the fun begins!) will emerge as you discover how to turn the obstacles that loom like giants before you, into life regenerating springboards for personal success.

Part Two (having laid a proper cognitive mindset foundation) builds on the previous section by introducing time-tested strategies used by many of the world's most successful men and women to accomplish great things (Sessions Seven through Nine).

A built-in goals program with powerful and easy to use exercises and inspirational instruction will assist you in developing your own personal blueprint for life success (Sessions Ten through Fifteen).

Fascinating real-life client stories (identity and details hidden to protect privacy) interwoven throughout will encourage and amaze as you discover that the problems people face are common to all of us, and that they can indeed be overcome by applying the principles outlined in this book.

Now that we've been introduced, let's head into the office to begin our first session.

Part One

Cognitive Boot Camp

(Putting the "C" in New Mind Synergy = CG^2)

"Give me a 'c'!"

$$NMS = CG^2$$

New Mind Synergy

SESSION ONE

WHERE DOES IT HURT?

Suffering has been stronger than all other teaching. . . . I have been bent and broken, but I hope into a better shape.

-Charles Dickens

A Pleasure Meeting You

Upon entering, you settle into (sitting, not lying down—this isn't Freudian psychoanalysis) the brown, cozy leather couch nestled comfortably next to the miniature forest of plants, fresh flowers, and ancient European oil paintings that line the mahogany encased bay window warmly accenting the interior of my office.

Once seated, we exchange pleasantries and spend a few moments becoming better acquainted. Gradually, the conversation shifts. I lean forward, intently listening as you painfully recount the failure that has driven you to seek my services. It is now that I learn why you are here, namely, where it hurts. This is important because your pain is fueling your desire for change.

The Common Threads of Human Hurting

I have had the privilege of working with individuals and families from all walks of life who encounter a broad range of painful personal struggles. Many of whom have courageously shared with me their story of tragedy and bitter disappointment, e.g., relationship failure; loss of a job or career; loss of a loved one; loss of reputation or self-respect; self-defeating behavior; battles with an addiction; or a total collapse of personal confidence. While the details of each situation are unique, nevertheless, common threads interweave the tapestry of our human experience with respect to feelings of emptiness and discouragement, and at times even hopelessness or despair.

Human Hurting as a Motivator

In virtually every case, the healing process begins when an individual first acknowledges his or her painful plight. Then, having acknowledged it as such, he or she successfully confronts the crucial decision as to how to best remedy the root cause and source of the pain.

Each person must ask him or herself this question: "Will I continue masking my pain by pretending to be someone or something that I am not?"

The beautiful thing about this book is that you will discover, perhaps for the first time, that it is okay to be you, just the way you are. You no longer need to hide from your past. Instead, you are invited to embrace it. By being your true, authentic self you can make progress more quickly and easily.

That is because the events of your life, both good and bad, serve as a foundation of experience far too precious and hard-earned to waste. The truth is, from your life experience, regardless of how difficult, you can move on to build a bright and exciting future.

Another question that individuals must ask themselves is: "Will I choose to medicate the pain that I feel by practicing an addiction?"

The problem with an addiction is that it numbs an individual further and further from reality. Consequently, an addiction represents little more than a failure to really grow, learn, and live.

Overwhelmingly, the most successful outcome occurs when an individual embraces his or her pain and draws from it every ounce of character and skill building life education possible. This is really the only true path to personal growth and inner healing.

Since you are here, chances are you have chosen this path for your life. That is great!

NO PAINS, NO GAINS. If little labour, little are our gains: Man's fortunes are according to his pains.

-Robert Herrick, 1650

The Gift of Pain

It may seem like an odd concept at first, but I invite you to begin thinking of your personal pain as a gift. Yes, a gift! Naturally, you might wonder how pain can be considered a gift.

Pain is an effective alert system. It is nature's way of highlighting the need for attention to an area of your mind, body, or spirit.

A Motto for Life

As a thirteen-year-old Pop Warner football player, residing in the sports-oriented community of Rancho Penasquitos, a suburb of San Diego, California, I recall how much I looked up to the Sun Devil high school football players donning muscle t-shirts that read, "No Pain, No Gain!" This was a reference to the demanding weightlifting workout schedule that characterized an important element of the community's serious and carefully crafted high school football training program. I doubt anyone, including myself, could have anticipated the profound effect this saying would have on me in years to come. In fact, it became a motto for life.

Upon reflecting, I can recall some very painful experiences. I am sure you can too. And yet, I am almost immediately aware of the fact that those very experiences were also the most formative in terms of my personal growth and development as a person. I realize now that the more painful the experience, the more I learned and grew as a result. Indeed, there is an element of pain that serves a very useful function.

Passing Lessons Along

Several months ago I pulled into a gas station parking lot after my daughter, Madison, age seven, alerted me to the fact that my son, Christopher, age three, had removed the safety belt straps from around his shoulders. Although we were in a hurry to arrive at our destination, I wanted to re-fasten the straps before continuing to drive. Perhaps you can relate to this scenario.

After tightening the straps, I slammed the back door of the car. There was just one problem. My thumb did not make it out of the way in time!

The next thing I heard was Madison asking, "Daddy, are you all right?" This was followed by a faint, curious, "Daddy are you going to cry?" The first question was sweet, the second, a challenge! Christopher was staring inquisitively, not quite sure what just happened.

Wincing in pain, I sat for a few moments holding back the tears. After all, as a dad, I had to maintain my macho bravado, right? While I did not end up crying (although if I had, it certainly would not have been the end of the world, as there is definitely a time and place for that—yes, even for a man), nevertheless, I experienced a throbbing sensation that lasted for several days.

As we continued to drive, I (as the ever-ready teacher) explained to my daughter the reason for pain and how it is nature's way of alerting us to a problem. She looked receptively, nodded in acknowledgment, and then referenced an experience she had a few months earlier when she also had slammed her finger in the classroom door (this seems to run in the family!). She asked, "Was it like that Daddy?" I replied, "Yes sweetheart, just like that."

The Hidden Danger of Remaining Numb

Some people cannot feel physical pain. The category of disorders which this falls under can be categorized as HSAN: Hereditary Sensory Autonomic Neuropathy. HSAN patients are exposed to a risk that most people do not have, the risk of *not feeling pain*. This is considered a risk factor for some fairly obvious reasons, namely, the inability to receive an alert that there may be something wrong medically that requires attention. It would be possible for someone with HSAN to literally bleed to death without ever knowing it!

In the scriptures, the Psalmist invites us to meditate on the fact that our bodies are "fearfully and wonderfully made" (Psalm. 139:14, NASV). This is true. Amazingly, our bodies alert us to physical, emotional, and spiritual issues so that we will act to obtain proper attention and care.

The Day Pain Entered My Life

I recall that on September 2, 1999, at a church conference in Shelbyville, Indiana, I was in need of direction and guidance for my life and the new counseling outreach ministry that I had recently founded. It was a deeply spiritual and moving conference, and one that I shall never forget.

An evangelist (an itty-bitty older gentleman with more hair than height) whom I had never met was in attendance. He was scheduled to speak that night. He had what is known in the church as "the gift of prophecy." That is, he received revelations from God often given as verbal messages to the intended recipient regarding various aspects of a person's life and future. As he was preaching, he turned my way. I quickly tried to duck behind the pew in front of me, but he was quicker. His eyes locked-in on me. "Oh no," I thought, "I'm pegged!"

Sure enough, he had a message for me.

His message went something like this: "You have been frustrated. You wonder what God is going to do with your life and ministry (this was true but I had not told this to a soul!). . . . You will have a compassionate ministry. . . . Your ministry will affect many lives. . . . Be patient and keep serving Him." To be truthful, although I believed him, I did not see this happening for me quite yet. At the time, I really did not see myself acting in any sort of extraordinarily compassionate way.

"What?" "Is there going to be a ministry of compassion for me?"

Then it dawned on me. Oh, no. If I was to have a compassionate counseling ministry, then I would have to go through some "stuff." Oh yes, that is exactly what this meant. "Oh, no" I thought. Oh yes!

I approached a couple of the elder ministers who were conducting the ordination ceremony and told them of my concerns and how I had interpreted this message. I declared, "This means I am going to have to go through some pain!" They replied, "Chris, do not be afraid! Embrace pain when it comes into your life."

Well, it happened all right. In fact, for the next several years that followed, I went through nothing but "stuff," of the "painful stuff" variety!

The Fruits of Pain

It would be several more years before the "compassionate ministry" portion of this prophecy would come into fruition. But now it has, in some remarkable and unexpected ways.

Today, I have the privilege of serving clients representing all walks of life, many of them in considerable pain.

I have also had the privilege of seeing clients pick up the pieces of their shattered lives, build beauty from ashes, and progress toward a triumphant new life of success, personal fulfillment, and peace.

Reflecting, I know it is the pain that I have personally walked through that has enabled me to assist my clients with far greater effectiveness than I would have had I not experienced my own personal baptism through the fires of pain.

Characteristics of Survivors of Pain

Over the years, I have observed eight key characteristics notably intrinsic to the men or women who move gracefully through pain and failure, exiting as butterflies from the cocoon's long, dark nights—fully formed and ready for flight. These characteristics are as follows: (*i*) *honesty*, especially with themselves; (*ii*) *personal responsibility*, they take ownership for their contributions to life's difficulties, instead of blaming others. They work hard in sessions and between sessions to develop greater self-esteem, applying useful self-help literature and exercises to their lives. Research shows that self-help does work; (*iii*) *positive attitude*, they learn to capture redeeming value in virtually everything; (*iv*) *spirit of forgiveness*, they do not harbor resentment and anger; (*v*) *vision* for their lives, through a process of self-analysis, they became aware of their true life's passion, and set-forth boldly with committed focus and perseverance to personally realize their vision for life success; (*vi*) *courage*, to go against the grain—silencing the voices of fear, friends, and family members who told them that they were crazy for breaking the mold of conformity, and for taking such a reckless risk in order to achieve their vision; (*vii*) *reliance on a mentor, group, or community of people* who graciously model and encourage personal transparence and life success; and finally, (*viii*) *faith* that change is possible. We must believe that change is possible in order to persevere.

By the way, belief that is born out of need is often the most powerful. I love the way the book *You Love Me, Don't Accept Me As I Am* (2006) puts it, "Knowledge alone of a path or activity will not necessarily trigger action, because it is not anchored in a need of the individual."

Personal Inventory

Please take a few moments to do a personal inventory of how these eight key characteristics either are, or are not, exemplified in your own personal experience. Is there anything preventing you from maintaining a similar mindset?

As you reflect, can you see how interrelated these characteristics are one to another?

Virtually all of these eight characteristics are represented in some form or fashion in the strategies to follow.

Every Adversity carries with it the seed of an equivalent or greater benefit.
-Napoleon Hill

SESSION TWO

COGNITIVE ROOTS OF FAILURE

The roots of education are bitter, but the fruit is sweet.

-Aristotle

I fully expect that somebody at this point might argue, "Chris, you are focusing too much on the 'down-and-out' side of things. I mean, come on, a whole session about 'pain', and now about the 'roots of failure'? Let's move on to what makes us successful already!"

However, according to this introductory quote by Aristotle, we see that bitter experiences provide a foundational component of our lives education. Therefore, pausing here to put things in proper perspective just may not be such a bad idea.

Is this to say that we can only learn by bitter experiences? I do not think so. In fact, it's great when we can learn life's lessons from those who have gone before us, as well as through positive and more pleasurable means. I am all for that!

I think Aristotle is saying that many of life's lessons require hard work, sometimes even brutal effort, to the point of being bitterly hard. They stem from difficulty and even unpleasant life experiences. Let's face it. Most of us can be pretty stubborn! Our human nature often will not listen until we are made to feel uncomfortable. Finally, being formed from the root, they are an essential predecessor to the resulting sweet fruit.

Biologically, sadness may be more instructive for the long haul.

-Eric Jensen

What Does Not Kill You Makes You Stronger!

You have probably heard the sayings, "What doesn't kill you makes you stronger," and "Hindsight is twenty-twenty," or perhaps you've heard someone say, "I used to think, say, or do this or that, but now I am much wiser." These are all perfect examples of the "sweet fruit" mentioned above.

Anytime we are educated by life's difficulty, and after applying what we have learned, can see positive results, we become living examples of Aristotle's sentiments as expressed in this session's opening quote.

Also implied by this quote is the contrast between *bitter* on one hand, and *sweet* on the other. Contrasting is a powerful literary device used to illustrate an authors or speakers point with maximum impact. It is likely that Aristotle did not have to stretch far to glean value from this reality in the physical world, as nature is full of contrasting elements that serve as profound object lessons.

How does this translate into the human experience? Namely, that we should not be alarmed, discouraged, or ashamed when we experience difficulty, because difficulty is an intrinsic element of our education—a prelude to the sweetness that life can potentially yield if we will but listen, learn, and apply the lessons.

The Fortunate Few

Most of us have met people who seem to breeze through life with ease and grace. We notice that they don't seem to inflict much harm on themselves. While certainly not immune from life's difficulty, they seem to manage it with relative grace. I have known a few such lucky souls.

My observation has been, and research seems to support, that these are people who are socially, emotionally, physically, and spiritually "operating on all cylinders." They are healthy in virtually every respect, resulting in an easier time of things. Oftentimes, they are more socially adept—fulfilling wants and needs equitably. Being unencumbered by emotional baggage allows them to remain free from over-asserting "self" as they go about getting their wants and needs met. Hence, they are well-liked and enjoy a rich and intimate experience with friends and family. They are emotionally healthy, and as a result, typically make good decisions. As a result of experiencing less social and emotional stress, they are physically healthier and maintain strong levels of energy for accomplishing tasks and enjoying life. Additionally, they are more spiritually centered, as if freedom in the social, emotional, and physical areas of life—via "clean cognitive hardware"—allows them to hear God's voice with greater clarity and respond with greater precision. Finally, they are prone to make thoughtful, logical, and evenly measured life decisions—resulting in a rewarding vocational experience and relatively strong financial standing.

While this variety of person is certainly to be admired and appreciated for their attributes, it is important to recognize that this does not characterize the experience of many.

The Common Person

Many people will struggle with depression, anxiety, a family breakup, loneliness, confusion, addictions, an inability to connect and form intimacy, vocational unhappiness, financial trouble, legal problems, a troubled or ill child, or any of a myriad of other issues at some point in their lives.

Let's face it. Life can be painful and difficult!

There are so many elements that can be potentially stacked against us that the chances of experiencing significant failure at some point in our lives are high. Just by breathing, by being alive, we are subject to this world's difficulty. It is all a part of the human condition.

Learn to Play Your Cards Well

Therefore, I want you to begin thinking less in terms of shame or embarrassment for your shortcomings and failures, and more in terms of the sweetness that emerges as a result of taking the cards you were dealt and learning to play them well—in order to obtain a more positive result. The remainder of this book will show you how.

The Wounded Healer

I have observed that people who draw from their inner resources of faith and strength of spirit to overcome obstacles often carry a profound breadth and depth of character. In turn, they are equipped to more effectively help their fellow man through the forest's dark night. For such, the bitterness of education yields a sweet fruit, much like a mature grape that is pressed to bring forth a rich and flavorful wine.

Failure Hit Close to Home

In my personal journey, I recognized that various issues were impeding my progress toward the things I really wanted in my life. Therefore, I began confronting issues head-on, until I achieved a resolution that seemed satisfactory. It was around this time that I discovered the power of setting goals.

The Synergistic Power of Goals

Upon reflecting, I realize that by strategically addressing my own personal challenges while simultaneously implementing the power of a well-formulated goals program, produced a much welcomed synergistic outcome. The word "synergy," repeated here for those who have skipped over the Preface and Introduction—they do exist you know!—comes from the ancient Greek term *syn-ergos*, which is used to describe the compounding phenomena of two or more agents working together, achieving considerably more than two single agents acting independently could achieve, and resulting in an end product that is greater than the sum of its parts.

As I resolved personal challenges, which I like to call "cognitive house cleaning," my goals and purpose in life became clear. As my goals and purpose became clear, personal issues seemed to more easily take care of themselves.

This could easily spark a debate similar to, "Which comes first, the chicken or the egg?" i.e., cognitive house cleaning or goals. Answer: It really does not matter!

Just as I can enjoy an omelet for breakfast, or a hearty serving of chicken soup for dinner, so I can enjoy the benefits of the end-product of strategically knocking out personal challenges, while simultaneously working toward my goals in life, and vice versa.

As I applied this approach with clients, they began making tremendous strides, gaining a sense of hope and purpose, realizing that they too can move forward to live more purposeful, dynamic, and rewarding lives.

Change at the Core

The reason this multi-modal (synergistic) approach (New Mind Synergy = CG2) to working with clients is so valuable (and has become the signature of my private practice), is because all-too-often, people move forward to accomplish things, while ignoring the all-important inner work necessary to achieve lasting success.

They start well, but become disillusioned when inner turmoil, amplified by the difficulty and stress which almost always accompanies any significant undertaking, enters the equation, and things eventually blow up in some way. Assigning themselves as hopeless cases, they likely drift into lives of silent desperation and mere survival, instead of what I term, "life-thrival."

The Danger of Apathy

Unfortunately, our culture is filled with people who suffer self-inflicted ills, such as forms of depression. Depression develops for a variety of reasons, and many times *not* a fault of the individual inflicted by it. However, depression defined as the chasm between ones present life and where that person's heart of hearts longs to be, can sometimes be the result of personal choices to remain stuck—all because an individual is content to allow the currents of life to carry them along the pathways of least resistance.

Content in their misery, or passively counting on a magic moment when everything will somehow work out (like a fool's gold hunt, the magic moment never emerges) they are not forging ahead and striving for personal growth and the achievement of positive goals for their life.

The laws of nature teach us that stagnancy, self-neglect, and the path of least resistance result in weakness, decay, and ultimately, death.

What happens to a plant once it stops growing? It atrophies. Similarly, what happens to a river that ceases to flow? It becomes stagnant.

In our culture today, the devastating effects of idleness are evident in an increasingly unsteady emotional profile among many children, teenagers, and young to middle-aged adults who have been trained to believe that life is about ease and pleasure, and void of any real meaning or higher purpose.

What Columbine Taught Us

In the wake of the tragic Columbine school massacre of 1999, I developed a workshop for families in response to the perceived need for parents to approach family life and parenting with a greater degree of intentionality. The workshop is entitled, "Foundations Four (4) Family Success."

Interwoven throughout the foundations of my workshop are powerful concepts I learned from a seminar conducted by Family Life Educator and Author, Gary Smalley (and later expounded upon in a more recent book, Smalley, et al, 2010). They include the notion that parents must engage their children by working together to discover their unique family identity (much like the mission statement of the preamble and laws of the United States Constitution provides national boundaries, a mission, and identity). Discovering a family identity involves a time of reflection, establishing a clearly written set of expressed values and rules of conduct, and a family mission statement. As Stephen Covey says, "The whole family can begin with the end in mind, a common purpose, a common vision."

These articles are intended to reflect the specific rules, boundaries, and guidelines that will govern the family's choices and actions. By the end of the workshop, the family will have started to create (this is an ongoing, evolving family growth process) a set of documents entitled, *Family Mission Statement*, and *Family Constitution*. They can frame and then hang these articles in a prominent place within their home.

What Our Youth Desperately Crave

Youth yearn for family cohesion, behavioral boundaries, clearly defined values, and a sense of life meaning and purpose—important elements increasingly snatched from the fabric of our culture over the past several decades—wherein *spiritual truth* and *moral absolutes* have progressively been usurped by an unfortunate trend towards *spiritual* and *moral meaninglessness*.

A family mission statement and constitution help foster an important sense of safety, trust, and self-esteem in both young children and teenagers alike. Young people begin to absolutely thrive as a result of being included in the drafting of a family charter.

Do you suppose that as co-creators of the family mission statement and constitution, children will actually adopt a greater sense of "ownership" and "buy-in" to the common interests and rules of the family? Could this inclusive framework really help prevent parent-child alienation, as well as an entire host of potential problems families often encounter through the pre-teen and teenage years? Research strongly supports this notion. That is why I still offer this workshop today. It has become the most popular family coaching program that I offer.

Fill It, or Fold!

As I studied the dynamics that led up to the events at Columbine, it became abundantly clear that if parents fail to foster within their children a clear sense of direction, meaning, and purpose, then destructive elements existent within our world will likely fill that void—typically, with undesirable and sometimes even tragic consequences.

Parents are charged with the responsibility of fostering healthy cognitive development and strong decision making abilities within their children. Let's face it. Children can learn life's lessons at an early age, while the price is relatively low, or similar lessons, only with heavier and potentially life-altering consequences, at later stages of development, well into adulthood.

What holds many people back is the fact that they were not properly trained while younger. Many twenty-, thirty-, and forty-something's are struggling to learn what they should have learned in grade school, middle school, and high school.

Cognitive immaturity results from inconsistent childhood discipline, lack of positive role modeling, and poor social skills training. Acting as children in grown-up bodies, many are ill-prepared to meet the demands of life in a responsible and productive manner.

The good news remains that even as an adult you *can* still learn and grow. While it is more difficult and painful to learn life's lessons in one's adult years, it is never too late. After all, that is why this book was written.

Let's Dive In

Now, let's dive into some of the more common cognitive roots of failure. Perhaps you can identify ways in which one or more of these roots have contributed to failure in your life.

Remember, the goal is not to get bogged down by the problems, i.e., stumbling blocks that we will highlight, but to use the insight learned as clues, informing your strategy in moving forward towards life recovery, and becoming your ultimate and best self.

Sessions Three and Four feature the dynamic science behind the remedies for such stumbling blocks, and together with Session Five, link practical and powerful strategies and techniques for destroying the cognitive roots of failure, and growing a healthy mind forest.

The Cognitive Roots of Failure

Some of the more common cognitive, thought-oriented roots of failure are as follows:

Addictions

Being addicted to something is often equated with being in prison. The reason is because an addiction strips a person of one of his or her most valuable possessions, freedom. It is impossible to be free, and enslaved by a destructive behavior or substance at the same time.

From seemingly insignificant compromises of your personal discipline and values, to full-blown addiction, the result is a diminished capacity to be fully present, fully alive, and fully connected to those around you.

An addiction makes it virtually impossible for the mind to function at an optimal level. Energy and electro-chemical resources within the mind that might otherwise surge to activate a positive, life giving, synergistic result, must now be diverted to help manage the crisis of consequence, shame, and guilt associated with the addiction cycle.

The psychoanalyst would of course argue that this is where the "id" (drive for pleasure), "ego" (moral sense, or sense of self), and "superego" (highly moral) come into conflict, stripping the mind of vital energy that could otherwise be focused more productively. This is true. A mind in conflict with itself is a mind preoccupied, and hence, depleted of mental vitality.

Addiction specialists often equate the development of an addiction as an attempt to numb one's self through *repression*, burying painful experiences and emotions, and *dissociation*, the defense that often accompanies the devastating and shaming effects of sexual and/ or physical abuse. Dissociation attempts to deny what is happening presently or what happened in the past, and elicits the distracting elements of imagination to do so.

The addicted person will often rationalize that he or she is somehow slowing more severe forms of self-destruction through alcohol and drug use, as opposed to taking the steps necessary to become truly healthy.

A primary component of recovery for the addicted individual includes both identifying and resolving sources of unhealthy shame and guilt, and reinforcing those processes that will limit their destructive effects.

The net result of an addictive thought process is that less of *you* is present, and less of *you* is truly alive and able to freely engage with those in your inner-circle.

Since the scientifically established premise of the Get Up! *Ultimate Life Recovery Program* is that change is indeed possible; you've now become fully aware that an addiction does not have to rule over, defeat, or control you.

Having a genetic predisposition to alcohol or drugs is no longer an excuse for remaining in the addiction cycle. Herein is presented an opportunity to change before it's too late.*

In addition to the potentially tremendous benefits which come from reading this book, please consult a trained addictions specialist near you if you are currently struggling with an addiction.

Clarity (lack of)

In Luke's gospel, chapter 14, and v. 28-32, Jesus asks,

"For which one of you, when he wants to build a tower, does not first sit down and calculate the cost, to see if he has enough to complete it? Otherwise, when he has laid a foundation and is not able to finish, all who observe it begin to ridicule him, saying, 'This man began to build and was not able to finish.' Or what king, when he sets out to meet another king in battle, will not first sit down and take counsel whether he is strong enough with ten thousand men to encounter the one coming against him with twenty thousand? Or else, while the other is still far away, he sends a delegation and asks terms of peace."

Oftentimes, we fail because we venture forth without clarity. Therefore, I often ask my clients, or members of an audience, "What is it that you truly want for your life?" Almost always the answer is the same, "happiness."

Happiness is certainly a very positive emotion to desire. After all, who does not want to be happy? The problem with such a vague response is that it lacks specificity, and therefore, clarity. It is only as I probe deeper that I learn more definitively what happiness represents to him or her.

It is amazing to me how many people drift through life without a clear and specific plan of action. Having only a vague idea of what they truly want out of life, and moving forward in a nonchalant and haphazard way, they experience very little positive results (and typically quite a few disastrous ones!), and become discouraged. Have you ever wondered if the unhappiness, emptiness, and boredom you might experience from day-to-day results from failing to engage a bigger vision for your life?

Options Awareness

Oftentimes, we are limited by our lack of cognitive awareness. We remain unaware of the myriad of options and resources available to us. Options limited, we become stuck and settle for less than what is truly possible. We fail to realize that a whole world, with virtually millions of options, is waiting.

This is why when I opened my private practice, I was so thankful for the years I had spent as a Clinical Social Worker (CSW). As a CSW, one of my chief tasks involved linking clients with available resources and services. Over time, this helped me understand the tremendous value of learning to think outside of the confines of a present circumstance, and to explore and help implement resources that could more effectively address client needs.

Become Perfectly Clear

It is essential that you invest time in understanding yourself, and your true goals and mission for living. Only once you have invested the time to become absolutely clear about what you truly want are you ready to take significant action. The reason for this is simply that anything worth accomplishing will be met with some degree of difficulty, and therefore, will naturally require proper planning and persistent effort. Otherwise, you might easily fall victim to defeat—as the examples of both the builder of the tower, and the king, so richly illustrate.

As entrepreneur, author, and coaching expert, Brian Tracy, says, "Casualness brings casualties" (Tracy, 2003).

Since you certainly do not want to become a casualty, it is imperative that you stop merely existing, become perfectly clear about what you truly want for your life, and start living. Remember, you only live once!

Codependence

Codependence is problematic for many.

It is impossible to be your best self when you settle for relationships that you know are sucking the life right out of you!

Most of us crave intimacy and the good feelings that come from being in a relationship with someone for whom we have affection. This is normal. However, when we remain in an unhealthy or abusive relationship (especially one that puts our personal safety, or that of our loved ones, at risk, or runs contrary to our life's goals, values, and best interests) because of emotional neediness, insecurity, fear of loneliness, fear of retribution, fear of embarrassment, fear of what others will think, or convenience, then we greatly limit ourselves.

Bargaining through a codependent relationship often travels along one or more of these lines: "I can't live without him or her"; "He or she needs me"; "What if no one else wants me?"; "I can't stand to be alone"; "What if I don't make it on my own?"; "He will be so angry and may try to hurt me"; "What if others laugh at me should I fail . . . again?"; "What will they say or think if I fail in this relationship?"; or "But I may have to go without nice things. . . . Life will be so hard!"

For some, the abuse suffered at the hands of an emotionally distant parent was the only time they felt a connection to that parent. It was anything but easy to endure. It hurt. But it felt better than being ignored!

When Mom or Dad was abusing, at least they were engaging the child while the abuse was taking place. In such cases, a semblance of intimacy is derived through being abused, and the pattern is then perpetuated by selecting similar dynamics in future relationships.

Our baseline stress level, what we would call a normal degree of stress, is not set for life. Life experiences can and do reset our brain's "stress thermostat" at a higher level, so that we experience higher levels of stress reactivity if we have been exposed to particularly intense or repeated stressors within a short time frame, or emotional trauma (Jensen, 2005).

Anyone who remains in a particular "state" (such as a stress state) for too long, potentially risks stabilizing that state within the nervous system. For instance, experiencing normal levels of conflict or stress in a relationship is not necessarily a problem. The problem develops when we fail to do anything about it—we allow the conflict and the stress state that goes with it to persist. The longer the state persists, the more reinforced and familiar it becomes to the nervous system. It becomes comfortable—home. It should then come as little surprise when we unwittingly seek that state out of familiarity or comfort (Jensen, 2005).

This dynamic of homeostasis ("home state," or more loosely referred to as, "comfort level") manifests as an attraction to, or increased comfort with, stressful, chaotic, or emotion-laden relationship experiences. This home state is that state to which we have become accustomed. Therefore, we choose it time and again, oftentimes without realizing why.

A person can get out of this abusive cycle by (*i*) weighing the cost of remaining in the relationship (seeing oneself as valuable is paramount here), (*ii*) working with a professional to obtain a greater degree of emotional health and strength, (*iii*) forming a support network, (*iv*) generating a plan of action or escape, and (*v*) desiring to begin living with a higher purpose in mind.

I have met many people who offer themselves at the altar of destructive relationships. They diminish their potential for growth and true freedom, and instead merely exist in a state of silent desperation. They later spend much of their lives thinking, "What if . . . ?" or "If only I had . . .!" Fill in the blank.

Fear of the unknown, of leaving the familiar, forms a powerful shackle. Manipulated by voices that say "you can't," or "I can't," can be overcome only by taking that first step. Then, as if alive for the first time, you discover that a whole new world is there for the taking, and that you *can* move forward towards something better.

If this describes you, my sincere hope is that you will tap into the courage that resides within you to break free and really begin living.

Dysthymia, Major Depression, and Anxiety

Dysthymia

On any given day, approximately twenty-five million Americans feel down in the dumps, and suffer some of the symptoms of depression.

Dysthymia is a milder, yet persistent, and often overlooked form of depression. It can be hard to identify, because, while the symptoms are similar, dysthymia is not as severe as major depression. However, these less severe symptoms often last for a period of two years or longer.

Dysthymia robs an individual of vitality and zest for life. The crispness and clarity necessary for making good decisions, as well as personal confidence, are stripped. In this low-grade depression, the color of life is snatched away.

Major Depression

Major depression is often debilitating. It is cunning in that the individual suffering with major depression is often the last to identify it as such. Some chief characteristics of major depression include: depressed mood, excessive guilt, fatigue or loss of energy, changes in sleep and/or appetite, excessive crying for no apparent reason, suicidal ideas, poor decision making ability, i.e., confusion, loss of interest in pleasurable things, and negative perceptions and thoughts.

Ultimately, depression ranges from mild, to moderate, to severe.

Hope alone is a powerful antidepressant.
-David Burns, M.D.

Anxiety

General anxiety disorder, obsessive compulsive disorder, post-traumatic stress disorder, panic attacks, phobias, and other forms of anxiety emerge for a variety of reasons. While the intent of this book is not to go in-depth into each of these, it may prove useful to keep in mind that they are physiologically and brain-based; they are environmentally triggered and/or nurtured; they are treatable. The information and exercises in this book should prove helpful towards managing depression and anxiety. Of course, any clinical disorder should be managed under the care of a mental health professional or physician.

I point these out because we live in a stress-filled culture in which there is diminished time for family and friends, resulting in decreased intimacy. Exercise, proper rest, healthy diet, and recreation compete with increased financial pressure—resulting in exhaustion, fear, and a general sense of personal loss.

These factors combine to create a cocktail for increased incidence of clinical disorders, and an imbalance in the physiological processes necessary for proper brain and body function.

A well-rounded and effective approach to maximizing your potential will include a careful consideration of these issues.

External Causes

You had little choice in the matter. Maybe you got clobbered by an act of nature, the recent economic downturn, someone else's irresponsibility, or just a really lousy boss. While not intrinsically a cognitive root of failure, an external event impacting a person in some profound way can play serious havoc on the mind.

And yet, it's all too easy to play the "blame game." You have some choices to make.

False Failure

> *Let the world know you as you are, not as you think you should be.*
> -Fanny Brice

False failure is a psychosocially rooted false perception of failure that occurs when an individual, despite doing quite well, is bombarded with messages to the contrary.

In some cases, our lives become pre-scripted by those well intentioned (and sometimes not so well intentioned) individuals, parents, extended family members, and friends who endeavor to control how our life is supposed to be lived—down to the very last detail. For example, the parent who pushes their son towards becoming a world class business mogul, when in reality, the son dislikes business; instead, he prefers painting and photography.

Unwittingly, we can fall into the trap of adopting other peoples' definition of success instead of our own. We assume an identity based on the expectations of others and become so embroiled in what we think we are supposed to do that we lose sight of our own definition of success and personal fulfillment.

In particularly persuasive, dogmatic, or shame-based cultures and subcultures, "wandering from the chosen path" can be met with intense and stifling guilt.

We wake up one day and have to face the fact that we have not met the expectations of others, but cannot figure out why. We see ourselves as internally defective, woefully undisciplined, or worse. We attempt to hide our pain by lying to ourselves and others. We live a double life.

Trapped between a belief about who we are supposed to be and who we really are, our growth becomes stunted: we live in conflict, become indecisive, our energy is fragmented, and we are rendered ineffective. Anytime we act like somebody that we are not, it strips away our vital energy, creativity, and confidence.

I love the way neuroscientist, author, and speaker, Dr. Caroline Leaf, puts it, "You can only be you. Who you are at the core will leak out, no matter how much you suppress it. . . . In order to sustain a consistent outlook and pattern, your thoughts, your words, your spirit and your actions must line up. That means when you say something that your brain doesn't 'believe' – if your statement isn't part of you on a cellular level – it is unsustainable" (Leaf, 2009).

We desperately need to get to the point where we say, "Enough is enough! No longer will I live my life according to other peoples' expectations. No longer will I define who I am by the measuring rods of others. Instead, I will determine the basis for my life's success."

"Your *own* gift is *more* than enough, and once you uncover that gift and its structure, you can walk in freedom, knowing yours is unlike anyone else's. . . . Your life experiences, the lessons you've learned, and your unique gift all combine, giving you the opportunity to walk into the future with unlimited potential to grow into your own success" (Leaf, 2009).

I knew you before I formed you in your mother's womb.

-Jeremiah 1:5

What is the bottom line? The bottom line is that you are unique, special, and gifted to contribute to the world and those around you in amazing ways. It is my hope that this program will assist you toward this endeavor.

Fear

This is a biggie!

There are two primary roots from which we operate—*love* and *fear*.

Fear often stems from childhood experiences. We grow up being told, "You had better," "You should," or conversely, "You cannot!" These messages become deeply imbedded within our subconscious mind.

Many of our decisions, being rooted in these fear-based messages, unwittingly determine our life's course, and alter our destiny. That is why it is essential that we take a thorough personal inventory and discover the ways in which fear influences our decisions and behavior on a daily basis, and then plan to make corrections.

At the present time, we live in a culture seemingly immersed in a fear-based mindset. With access to images of war, violence, natural disasters, poverty, and economic woes streaming 24/7 into our homes, and with so many people losing their jobs and sense of economic security, it is as if a wave of fear has swept through and imbedded itself within the collective mind of our culture. It could easily become a paralyzing fear if we are not careful.

Fear is the opposite of love. Love always hopes and embraces possibility. Therefore, it is essential that we counteract fear by beating it back with goal-oriented thinking, creativity, and a hearty appreciation for what is truly possible in each of our lives. We need to avail ourselves of the myriads of untapped opportunities for greatness all around us. This book is dedicated to helping you discover the way.

Grief (stuck in)

There is no pain as great as the memory of joy in present grief.

-Aeschylus, founder of Greek Trajedy

Grief is an emotional response to loss. However, becoming "stuck" in grief, what is often referred to as "complicated grief," presents a very real stumbling block for many.

Perhaps you are familiar with the term, "stages of grief?" In her 1969 book, *On Death and Dying*, Elisabeth Kubler-Ross introduced a model commonly known as the five stages of grief, including: (*i*) Denial, (*ii*) Anger, (*iii*) Bargaining, (*iv*) Depression, and (*v*) Acceptance.

While the grief process may not always be as neat and clean as 1-5, this model has provided a realistic and much welcomed framework for better understanding the stages through which most people journey en route towards successful resolution of grief.

This model is recognized and used by many mental health professionals to this day. Some models expand the stages into six (6) or seven (7), including such issues as "guilt," "life reorganization," and "recovery," etc. while maintaining much of the basic structure as that established by Kubler-Ross.

At any given point, a person can become stuck in one of the above identified stages of grief. In such cases, there exists a failure to work through to resolution, potentially resulting in a host of difficulties in moving forward with life in any real meaningful way.

While an extensive handling of this subject is beyond the scope of this book, and grief issues are generally best handled under the care of a competent therapist, it is my personal belief that the strategies and techniques outlined in this book can play an important role in one's ability to progress through grief in an effective and healthy manner.

Learning Problems

Learning problems such as, general learning, ADD, ADHD, and a variety of other cognitively centered difficulties (for ADD and ADHD, this especially includes the central nervous system) can undermine confidence, breed confusion, fear, and even self-loathing.

Many adults struggle with poor self-esteem, and can point to a learning difficulty as the root cause for their failure at a variety of life endeavors.

According to the Data Accountability Center, Part B Child Count 2008, nearly 2.5 million students are currently receiving special education services for learning disabilities in the United States. Forty-three percent of students receiving special education services through the public schools meet criteria consistent with a learning disability.

Also, 25% of students with a learning disability drop out of high school, versus 9.4% of students in the general population, and 61% of students with a learning disorder graduate from high school with a regular diploma, versus 87.6% of students in the general population—according to the 25th annual report to congress, U.S. Department of Education.

Clearly, something must be done to address the staggering needs represented by so many of our nation's young people, as well as adults suffering with learning difficulties.

Fortunately, educational therapists now have a better understanding of learning difficulties and the techniques that are most useful in strengthening a student's ability to become a strong and independent thinker.

Mediated, Socratic methods of learning seem to be the best approach. However, this particular style of education is often underutilized in public schools. We need to find a way to expand community-based educational therapy program availability so that more students can *learn to think*, as opposed to *passively receiving information*.

The good news is that change is possible, regardless of the age of the student. The brain is a dynamic, adaptive, ever-evolving bundle of potential at any age—it is never too late!

There are a variety of fantastic programs nationwide that address learning issues. The National Institute for Learning Disabilities (NILD) is an organization for which I have a particular fondness. NILD is committed to helping individuals become strong independent thinkers.

Perfectionism

Like many nervous tendencies, perfectionism is oftentimes rooted in fear, e.g., fear of being out of control. It is a way of coping with past or current feelings of insecurity about oneself or some particularly stressful or unsettling aspect of one's environment.

Perfectionists need to have everything lined up perfectly before they will step-out and launch something adventurous and new. However, the reality of life is that circumstances hardly ever line up perfectly. Perfectionists can often be found waiting at the starting line of life, hoping for better conditions—*tomorrow*.

This reminds me of a time when, as a boy, I was enjoying the day with my family at San Diego's Mission Beach. My older brother and I had wandered down the boardwalk in search of adventure, and girls I am sure! Before long, we happened upon a group of older ruffians urging us to buy a bicycle for a mere $20.00. They described the brand name bicycle in elaborate and attractive detail, stating, "It has a shiny chrome-dipped racing frame, matching brushed alloy wheels, three piece pedal cranks, and ultra-lightweight racing handlebars." It sounded really nice!

Was there a catch? Yes! The bicycle, they claimed, was at a friend's house. To buy it we would have to pay them $20.00 in advance, and they would retrieve the bike and deliver it to us in the same location.

Although this sounded like an odd way to do business, nevertheless, our excitement being overshadowed by only our naïveté, we proceeded to rush over and ask our mom for the money to purchase the bike.

She then proceeded to give us a lecture, saying, "If something sounds too good to be true, then it probably is." She was right!

What can we take from this?

Nothing worth having is ever obtained without paying a price. When something lines up too easily, we must ask ourselves, "Why is this so easy?", and "What is the catch?"

That is not to say that some good things don't just fall into our laps from time to time. They do. When this happens, we are wise to grab hold of them and cease the moment. However, in most cases, the things in life truly worth having, and keeping, come as a result of hard work and persistent effort. They do not just magically appear to us. Additionally, circumstances rarely ever line up perfectly.

Success loves risk takers, and rewards them accordingly. The paradox of life is curious, in that, the more we seek security, the more it alludes us.

-Brian Tracy

Perfectionists falter because they either do not launch, or they stop an endeavor when obstacles appear. Perfectionists need to learn to deal with ambiguity and adversity, instead of hiding in a cocoon of sameness, comfort, and convenience.

In terms of letting go of fear and insecurity, the initial launching steps are oftentimes the toughest. However, once the initial steps are made, watch out, the perfectionist is going to get it right!

Dr. Christopher R. Miller

The Deeper Roots of Perfectionism

Before leaving this section, we need to address the fact that perfectionists often believe that they must earn love and approval by being exceptional. Many perfectionists grew up in a home wherein one or both parents failed to communicate approval and unconditional love independent of performance. People can be admired and respected—but not loved—for their performance and accomplishments.

To care for someone, we must know them for who they truly are as a human being—this includes their pain and shortcomings, as well as their positive qualities. After all, "brokenness" is essential to being human.

One of the primary tenets of cognitive therapy is that all human beings are inherently broken and flawed. We constantly battle these flaws in an effort to become the person we think we *should* be. Nevertheless, our brokenness and shortcomings can become a source of strength once we confront and accept them. When we hide our shortcomings in shame, they eat away at us, rob us of joy, and cause us to isolate from others (Burns, 1993).

Meet Alice

I am currently working with a client who suffered an extremely difficult childhood. Her father was out of the picture, and her mother was often gone from home—drinking, and leaving her (since age 3) and her sister to make due all on their own. Alice recalls, "We often ate stale bread, cheese, and cereal, and drank state provided milk (from powder), because that was often all there was to eat throughout the day." She recalls that her sister, two years her senior, use to hit and verbally abuse her. With tears she recalls that one day her mother dropped her off at a woman's house (whom she had never before met) and did not return for a year. This woman use to spit on her and hit her. In virtually every way, her childhood was rotten, stressful, and impoverished.

In addition to a variety of other issues that we have addressed over this past year (as perfectionists often manifest symptoms of anxiety and obsessive compulsive behavior, via the need to control and bring stability to an otherwise uncontrollable or scary life situation), Alice's tendency to isolate from others presents a very real threat to her psychological health and well-being. Therefore, this issue has now become a primary focus of treatment. Alice admits, "I do not like talking with [getting close to] others because I feel they would not accept me if they knew of my shameful past." I have discovered that many people think this way. Currently we are going through the *Ten Days to Self-Esteem* workbook by David Burns, M.D. My hope is that Alice can confront, accept, and even embrace her past. As this will allow her to open-up and experience intimacy with others.

Meet Jerry

I love the story that Dr. Burns (1993) writes about a very successful businessman named Jerry who moved to Philadelphia from Detroit and who always suffered from depression, from shyness and nervousness around people, and from marital unhappiness. Dr. Burns writes, "Jerry came from a blue-collar family. His parents were German immigrants, and his father was a tough disciplinarian. No matter what Jerry achieved in school, it never seemed quite good enough. For example, if he got straight A's, his father would tell him to make sure he kept it up, instead of telling him how proud he felt. Although Jerry was a model student and a good son, he always felt inadequate and lonely. As far back as he could remember he felt nervous and uncomfortable around other people— including his classmates and family. He was ashamed to admit how he felt, so he kept it a secret. . . . He was convinced that people would look down on him if they knew how weak and defective he felt."

Jerry had taken a small business on the verge of bankruptcy and worked hard to turn it around. The business prospered and was eventually listed on the American Stock Exchange. He married a beautiful woman, lived in a fancy house, and was financially secure. Yet, in spite of his success, Jerry felt tense and anxious most of the time. In fact, work was the only place that he felt comfortable and in control. Outside of work, social situations were awkward, and Jerry even found it hard to be around his wife and family. He had very little self-esteem and rarely experienced any real satisfaction from his accomplishments.

Dr. Burns and his team came up with an exercise in an effort to help Jerry. The exercise was for Jerry to ride on the subway for an hour or two and after introducing himself and starting a conversation with at least ten people, he was to tell them of his insecurities, and that, although he was a successful businessman, he never really felt much like a success in life because he was terribly anxious and felt inferior to others. He could also admit to them that he has tried for years to hide his feelings from others for fear of what they might think. Finally, he could tell them that as of today, he'd decided to stop keeping it a secret and to begin simply telling people the truth about what he was really like.

At first, Jerry protested the assignment. He then agreed to it. The rest of the story goes on to recount how Jerry was met with compassionate and friendly responses from the other people on the subway. In fact, some of the people with whom he shared were dealing with difficulty in their lives, and shared too.

According to the story, Jerry reported that this was one of the first times in his life that he ever felt close to people, like a member of the human race. His nervousness disappeared, and he felt free to be himself and to connect with other people. He suddenly felt like he had something to offer, a way to form a bond.

Dr. Burns then goes on to write: "When we discover new ideas that are very important, they often come in the form of paradoxes. The paradox for Jerry was that his weakness, which he had spent his entire life trying to hide, had suddenly become his greatest asset. . . . The problem was the shame that Jerry felt, not the imperfections. Once he exposed his weakness to the light of day, as opposed to hiding it in the dark, it became his greatest source of strength."

Connecting and the Western Culture

And so it is with us. In our Western culture, which suggests that we must achieve as much as possible and aspire to perfection in life to be considered acceptable and lovable, many of us have come to believe that we cannot allow others to know who we *really* are. After all, we must be strong, and everything must be going perfectly okay, otherwise we fear being looked down upon. We reason that if they truly know us, they will reject us.

We need to move beyond this kind of thinking in order to experience true intimacy with others. Just imagine how freeing it would be to open-up about ourselves and leave the shame behind—all for the purpose of truly connecting with others in a meaningful way. How might this impact our psychological well-being? How might this impact the quality of our lives?

Psychoemotional Drag

Many people carry a plethora of negative memories and thought patterns, and the accompanying emotions that have built up over the years, that reside within their brain. I call this "psychoemotional drag."

Your brain is made of nerve cells. Thoughts, information, experiences, and memories are not just some ethereal or mystical phenomena. Instead, they form actual physical properties, similar to branches of a tree. Dr. Leaf writes, "Every thought makes up one of these nerve cells, with memories and other information growing off of it – the branches of the tree" (2009).

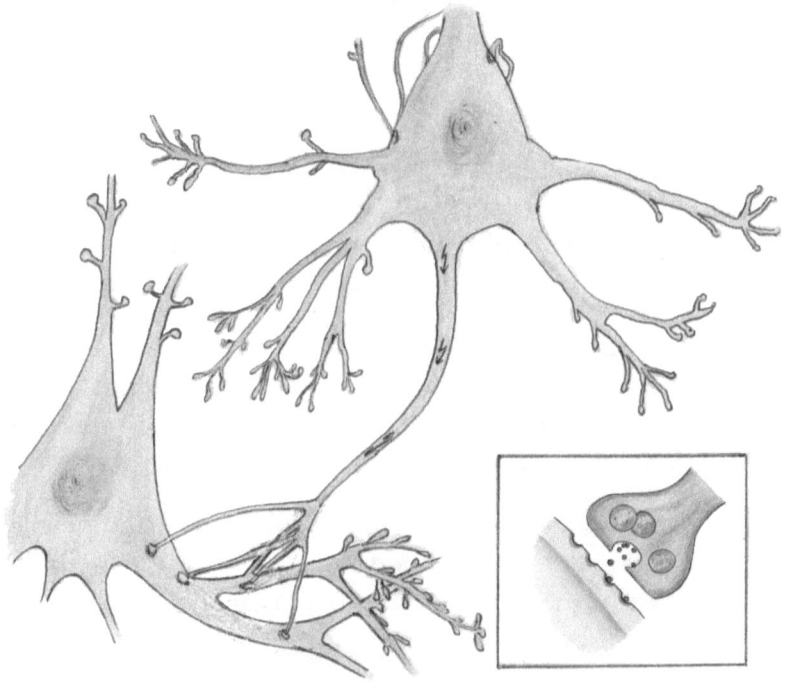

A signal transmitting down an axon to the cell body and dendrites (branches) of the next cell. Focus-frame, lower right, reveals this neurotransmission and reception of molecules at the synaptic level.

Everything you have ever experienced with your five senses (taste, touch, smell, hearing, and seeing), together with each thought you have ever had, is recorded and stored within your brain, wherein a new nerve cell branch is formed. Since your brain, like a computer, maintains an active filing system (a major difference is that your brain saves everything, without the need to push "save!"), every new experience and thought is stored on this neuronal super hard drive located within your subconscious mind.

Every time you experience something even remotely similar to a prior experience already stored there, your brain makes the connection and reacts in some way, i.e., favorably if the prior experience was interpreted by you as positive, and unfavorably if the prior experience was interpreted by you as negative.

Therefore, if you are not careful how you analyze incoming data, you may wind up misinterpreting a new event or situation. That is why it is possible to overreact, feel stress, or form a negative thought when encountering a situation that may not necessarily warrant such a response.

When this occurs, not only are you robbing yourself of an opportunity to react positively and form a new and more positive thought strand, but you are reinforcing and building upon the negativity that already exists as a very real part of your brains neuronal makeup.

A person who has suffered trauma, abuse, or any one of a number of painful and disappointing life experiences, but who has not been able to fully process or resolve it in a positive way, is potentially a psychoemotional drag candidate.

Every experience stored in the brain influences your thoughts, behavior, life choices, energy level, and mood far more than you may realize. Neuroscience has demonstrated that inflammation and swelling center around areas of the brain where unresolved emotional issues exist, thus impeding the balance of electro-chemical activity necessary to maintain a smooth and stable thought flow. This being the case, it becomes easier to interpret life events in a negative way, as the filters of interpretation are "toxic," and need to be made whole.

The good news is that the brain is equipped with a mechanism for both managing and destroying built up negativity. I call this the brain's "seek-and-destroy" mechanism (SDM).

Sessions Three through Five are devoted to helping you more fully understand and engage this amazing resource as you journey towards developing optimal cognitive functioning.

We need to clear our mind of unprocessed emotional baggage so that we can move through life with greater grace, ease, and fluidity.

Self Sabotage

Self sabotage is a dangerous and often hard to perceive psychological root of failure. Individuals who sabotage themselves crave messing everything up just so they can start all over again. They are addicted to the rush of being in a "one down" position, of starting over and reexperiencing the thrill of the chase. Their homeostatic maintainer, fancy words for *same state* or *comfort zone* as discussed previously, is set at: Impoverished and Happy Searching, Again.

Brooke's Story

When Brooke was a child her family moved to a new town or city approximately every one or two years. Her father was in the military. Brooke had always adored her father, but recalled feeling enormously sad when duty forced him to be gone from home for months at a time. Although her mother tried very hard and was basically a good wife and mother, she suffered chronic bouts of depression, which meant she was emotionally unavailable to Brooke a significant portion of the time.

Brooke recalled how many times after just becoming established and comfortable with her new surroundings, e.g., school, fellow students, and neighborhood friends, she would get the announcement from her mother—usually after school over a few of her favorite chocolate chip cookies and a glass of cold milk—"We are moving!" Brooke knew it would soon be time to begin again, *again*.

As an account executive for an internet-based financial services corporation, Brooke enjoyed tremendous work, schedule, and travel flexibility. She was free to move about the country, travel internationally and basically set her own schedule. She had enjoyed this lifestyle for many years.

However, a few years ago she realized that she had been running from commitment for nearly all of her life, e.g., she had never been in a relationship lasting for more than two years and had difficulty settling down within a community. She struggled with intense loneliness and feared she might someday die a "depressed and lonely old lady."

In a session late one summer afternoon, rather insightfully, she recalled, "Every time I think I want to settle in a place, I find something that I don't like, and the relationships I have managed to build come to an abrupt end. . . . I know the constant moving as a child has had a significant impact on my ability to 'dig-deep' and settle myself within relationships [relationships specifically, and social development more broadly]. It essentially modeled for me that I really do not have to work through issues that surface in the normal course of life. After all, change was bound to be just beyond the horizon, and probably sooner rather than later."

Brooke managed to amass a plethora of unpaid parking violation and library fines in various cities, and had bailed on leases for two different apartments in two separate cities (not to mention a host of damaged relationships in which resolution was never quite achieved—ouch!). Brooke lacked stability and maturity, and she knew it. As the saying goes, "a rolling stone gathers no moss."

This was Brooke—well intentioned, but moving too quickly to see projects, problems, and social issues through to constructive ends.

Brooke recounted, "I have always had this insatiable yearning to start something new." This was no surprise to me, because her homeostatic maintainer was very clearly set at "rebuild." And as a result of her tendency to become easily bored, Brooke always had lots of great projects and ideas (she was the best of visionaries) in the works, but with a less than an impressive project completion percentage.

Therefore, it came as no surprise when she described becoming confused about what she really wanted once the initial enthusiasm with which she started a project or venture began to wane. Becoming bored she would decide to quit and start something new.

Brooke recalls, "I didn't realize how I was behaving. This tendency shrouded itself by finding something I didn't like, and then creating an excuse to move on, to make a change, or to sabotage what I had in order to experience what I was used to, i.e., the thrill and rush of starting anew. Since I was used to adapting, this was usually not a problem for me."

When I first got this case I was blown away, because I could identify with Brooke on so many levels. Although much of what Brooke experienced was unique to her, and very different than anything I had ever experienced, I can still recall the enthusiasm with which I shared the principles and strategies that are now outlined in this book. They served as an invaluable anchor in my life, and I was sure they could help her as well. Like discovering a cool oasis amidst the hot, dry desert, Brooke drank in (dove in is more like it!) the New Mind Synergy strategies and techniques, and began applying them to her life in a very focused and determined way.

While Brooke's journey has certainly not been easy (consisting of a few challenges, twists, and turns along the way) she continues to make significant progress, i.e., she recently purchased a home, is dating someone seriously, and has anchored herself within a community. Her future has never looked more promising.

Meet Stan

Another example of self-sabotage is reflected in the experience of a former, short-term client—an actor who we will call, "Stan." Upon coming to see me, Stan revealed, "My whole life I have hated myself. If someone said something good about me, I immediately rejected it." He continued, "The more I was criticized, the more comfortable I felt. . . . If I experienced something good, such as, securing the leading role in a play, or enthusiastic applause after a performance, then I had to go and mess it up by drinking or using drugs until I felt lousy again."

While growing up, Stan's parents never told him that he was loved. In fact, they criticized him routinely. As a result, Stan rejected the accolades and acceptance of others, and any sort of good feelings that were not rooted in drugs and alcohol.

Stan's substance abuse issues subsequently led to the loss of a teaching position at a prestigious performing arts college, and the loss of numerous significant relationships. His health declining, and near financial ruin, Stan made the decision to reach out for help.

As Stan grappled to come to terms with such devastating losses, he eventually realized that for most of his life, he has been afraid of the rejection he feared might result if he were to allow someone into his life in a deep and personal way. Used to feeling lousy, he even sabotaged the career that for many years had meant so much to him. In his heart of hearts, Stan yearned for something better.

I made the decision to refer Stan to an inpatient treatment facility where he could receive medical intervention, group therapy, and intensive education about recovery from addiction. He has since graduated from the program. Last I heard, Stan continues to work hard towards his recovery by working with a sponsor, attending daily twelve-step meetings, and has remained clean and sober.

We Become What We Reinforce

Research shows that repeated or intense thoughts, behaviors, emotions, and life experiences actually form like physical characteristics within the brains neural circuitry, wherein the physical characteristics of brain neurons mirror a person's experience.

Every time a certain behavior is practiced it is reinforced and becomes stronger, as neural brain circuitry is grouped with like kind, forming a significant and increasingly influential thought-cluster. When this occurs, a person's "home"-state is set at a constant threshold, and he or she will do everything in his or her power to ensure that in some way, shape, or form, that certain place of comfort is maintained.

However, change requires that we begin to operate outside of this comfort zone. Therefore, change, by its very nature, is never easy!

That is why it takes conscious, intentional, and focused effort to change a negative pattern. The good news is that it can be done. The aim of Get Up! New Mind Synergy is to show you how.

Uni-dimensional Failure

Uni-dimensional failure means defining one's success in singular terms, for example, by the size of one's bank account. Only *one* thing really matters to the uni-dimensionally defined individual.

The problem here (besides having narrow vision) is that when the *one* (all- consuming) aspect of the uni-dimensionally defined person's life comes crashing down, he or she falls with it!

For the uni-dimensionally defined person, life becomes about control at all cost. Much the same as the instability of the proverbial three-legged barstool, this person unconsciously (or sometimes consciously) realizes that they are but a good swift kick away from sudden and total disaster!

Unforgiveness

> *To be wronged is nothing unless you continue to remember it.*
>
> -Confucius

The mere mention of the subject of unforgiveness evokes emotions in many people because it often carries with it painful thoughts, memories, and feelings of having been hurt by another person.

I will admit that it is difficult for me to write about this subject. It's not that I personally feel unforgiveness towards anybody. I am fortunate, in that, I do not. But because it is a humbling task for me to invite another person to forgive, especially when they have been deeply hurt by somebody in their life.

Truthfully, it is against human nature to forgive when we have been injured by another. And yet, it is essential for life, health, and vitality.

Devastating and life-altering consequences result when people harbor resentment, e.g., problems with blood pressure, heart, respiratory, and skin; depression; violent outbursts; anxiety; substance abuse; and diminished personal effectiveness all follow closely resentment's trail.

It is impossible to be our best and most vibrant self when we harbor resentment, bitterness, and anger towards someone else. As by nature these represent negative and destructive feelings.

What makes it easier for me to talk with people about this often painful and emotion-laden subject is the realization that in the end, the only one really hurt by harboring such feelings is their carrier.

Forgiveness releases a powerful chemical in the brain called *oxytocin*. (OX-ee-toe-sin) is a peptide also known as the "commitment molecule." It is released during sex and pregnancy and influences pair bonding. Females have more than males (Jensen, 2005).

Oxytocin is also released in response to attitudes, thoughts, and feelings of love, compassion, helpfulness, and the like. It has a powerful healing effect, and virtually melts away (into gas, literally!) the negative strands of resentment that once held a person captive (Leaf, 2009).

The goal is to maximize the brain's seek-and-destroy mechanism by better managing our negative thoughts, while building in plenty of loving, healthy, and positive thoughts via spiritual experiences and increased social connectedness.

Holding on to anger is like grasping a hot coal with the intent of throwing it at someone else; you are the one who gets burned.
-Buddha

Victim Mentality

Sometimes I meet people who play the victim role. They become befuddled and blame others when adverse circumstances arise. They do themselves a disservice by forgetting that life, by nature, is quite difficult, since others may not always cooperate with their plans.

The victim is almost always unhappy and feels beat down by life, choosing to operate under the paradigm of "external locus of control," as opposed to that of "internal locus of control."

External and internal locus of control are terms often used within the fields of counseling, psychotherapy, and coaching to describe an individual's basic disposition towards life. A person is either outwardly focused and other-determined, e.g., blaming circumstances and others for their own personal failure and misery, or internally focused and self-determined, e.g., maintaining an attitude that says, "the buck stops here," and taking responsibility for their own life and happiness.

The former are blaming, disempowered, ineffective, and negative about life and others; the latter are powerful, effective, and positive people.

Externally driven people have things happen *to* them, and thus, remain "victims" of circumstance. Conversely, internally driven people *create* their own circumstances.

In my observation (and perhaps you have observed this as well), it seems that victims are always having negative things happen to them. It is as if they have sent an "attack me" command out into the cosmos—the galactic macro-system that appears only all too willing to cooperate with their demands.

Victims attract negativity to themselves by virtue of their pessimistic attitude and orientation towards life. Their dance with the universe is unfriendly, resulting in negative attraction.

Victims are sick more often, get into more accidents, and generally have a difficult time with almost everything they endeavor to do. They send negative energy into the world, and they get back exactly what they are disposed to have in return.

Victims are often lonely. By being negative, blame-oriented, and by giving their power to others, they fail to attract people to themselves. By being other-determined and externally set, they are often bitter and resentful of others who have "wronged" them.

Unable to move beyond the bitterness, they suffer a myriad of health problems (as described in the previous section, *Unforgiveness*). Through their anger and self-victimization, they essentially ruin themselves.

Instead of taking responsibility and "reframing" (a technique we will get into more in Session Eleven) adversity as an opportunity for personal growth or a chance to see the "cloud's silver-lining," they shrink in despair and resentment for their perceived misfortune.

The victim role is often associated with codependency, as somewhere along the line, this tendency developed within the individual as a coping mechanism—remaining effective for a period of time. However, like all unhealthy coping mechanisms, the victim role has an expiration date, after which it becomes increasingly destructive.

Playing the victim role is a choice. It can be overcome by realizing that what once worked can no longer deliver. New choices must be made, and a new attitude and orientation to life must be formed.

People are attracted to positivity, success, and effectiveness.

Are you externally or internally driven?

Emotional Factors in Cognition

> *Emotion turning back on itself, and not leading on to thought or action, is the element of madness.*
>
> -John Sterling

The word "emotion" comes from the Latin *emovere* (*e* = away, *movere* = to move), meaning to move out of or to agitate. The root of this word is closely tied to *motivation.* Both indicate action. Such action is related to an individual's goals, so that essentially, motivation is action in pursuit of a goal (Howard, 2000).

This helps us better understand that emotion is action resulting from circumstances that either enhance or threaten a goal. Therefore, to the degree that I am motivated, I am pursuing a goal; to the degree that I am emotional, I perceive a threat to my goal (negative emotion), or significant progress toward my goal (positive emotion) (Howard, 2000).

"What does this mean to me?" you might ask.

It simply demonstrates the effects of motivation and goals on your emotional state. More specifically, it serves to highlight action versus inaction, and powerfulness (in happily, successfully, and confidently moving toward your goals) versus powerlessness (generating fear and emotional negativity whenever you are disconnected from what it is that you truly want for your life).

For now, it is important that you understand the interrelationship of thoughts and behavior (actions) and emotions.

Then, as we transition into Part Two (goals), this information will serve as a natural bridge between the cognitive portion (Part One) and goals portion (Part Two) of the books New Mind Synergy formula for success, NMS = CG2.

A Further Illustration of How Our Emotions Affect Us

> *The first funeral I ever attended was also my first introduction to the fragrance of gardenias. The nearness of gardenias still filters an event with a melancholy element.*

> -Joseph Ledoux

Meet Norma (this is a fictitious illustration, not an actual client)

Norma, a client services representative for a mid-sized insurance company, walks into her co-worker Bill's office hoping to obtain crucial account information before making an important telephone call to one of her clients. Upon entering, she immediately detects a strong whiff of black licorice permeating the air. Her colleague has apparently rediscovered his passion for black licorice, and eats it by the handful as a snack in between meals. Bill likely has no idea that Norma's ex-boyfriend absolutely loves black licorice, and ate it almost constantly while they were dating.

Unfortunately, her ex-boyfriend was cruelly abusive to her, and she suffered emotionally for several years as a result. Now upon smelling the black licorice (something quite benign), her mind quickly goes to unpleasant memories of her ex. Suddenly her brain has started to connect the smell of licorice with painful memory branches and negative

45

thought-clusters formerly lying dormant within the neural circuitry of her mind.

Norma proceeds to ask Bill for the account information, when suddenly she experiences a flood of negative thoughts and emotions. Her mood is beginning to slip.

Before entering Bill's office, Norma was having a good morning. But now her senses are starting to connect with neuronal branches of prior sensory experiences. Like a pinball, her thoughts now ricochet from memory to memory, and from thought-cluster to thought-cluster. Her brain is becoming saturated with negativity. She feels herself becoming depressed.

You might ask, "All of this because of the smell of black licorice?" Yes! This is an example of just how easily negative thoughts can be produced when one of our senses makes even an innocent connection with a negative memory.

But hang on a second—a moment of choice now emerges. There is still hope for a positive outcome for Norma! The brain sends and receives chemicals through what are called brain synapses. Neuroscientists often refer to brain synapses as the point wherein choices are made. At the moment of choice, the synapse will activate an electro-chemical reaction in accordance with a choice, thought, or interpretation of an event. A positive choice, thought, or interpretation increases the likelihood of a balanced, and therefore, positive electro-chemical reaction—which assists in forming new, healthy neuronal tree branches—adding health to the forest of the brain. Conversely, a negative choice, thought, or interpretation releases an unbalanced, and therefore, negative electro-chemical reaction—which assists in forming new, unhealthy neuronal tree branches—adding "toxicity" to the "forest" of the brain.

Norma can choose to allow the negative downward slide, or she can choose to counteract it with positivity—by rehearsing the truth about who she really is—her goals, potential, and enormous value as a woman. If she chooses the latter, healthier branches related to her past will begin to form, essentially melting away the negative thought-clusters over time. The choice is now hers!

Hopefully you can now begin to see how forming an abundance of healthy neuronal "trees of the mind" can have a compounding effect. It assists a person with the resources to increase the likelihood of interpreting daily events in a more positive way.

If this one example of a simple smell produced by something as seemingly insignificant as black licorice can create such emotional chaos, then just imagine with all the thousands of bits of information coming to us daily, and being interpreted by our senses, just how important it is that we guard our minds and thoughts, as well as pro-actively nurture a healthy mind forest.

Just imagine the result if Norma were to let her thoughts cascade further out of control. Who knows where she might end up? Might she be found eating black licorice with her ex? It happens all the time!

It is also important to keep in mind that various body regulating mechanisms, such as diet (Kolata, 1976), circadian rhythm (sleep), and hormonal levels (Kimura & Hampson, 1990, April), and to some degree, genetic vulnerability (J. G. Thompson, 1988) contribute to our emotional state as well.

Meet Tom (this is a fictitious illustration, not an actual client)

Another example is taken from the life of Tom. Tom was driving down the road with his family on a peaceful Sunday afternoon, when all of a sudden a car zoomed in front of him and cut him off.

Fortunately, Tom and his family did not wreck their car, nor did Tom think what appeared to be a careless miscalculation on the part of the other driver was an intentional act of aggression.

Regardless, he began to feel anger boil-up inside, a clear sign that his fight or flight responses were activated.

Now, a moment of choice!

Even though his wife was on his right, and two small girls were in the back seat, he sped up. For a split second he even thought to himself, "This is wrong. I should not react like this!" However, he chose to do so anyway.

He finally caught up to the driver in the other car, rolled down his wife's window, and started to read the guy the riot act!

It was not long before the two drivers began to fist fight.

Tom was thrown into the road and almost hit by a passing car!

During the fight, Tom's little girls were in the back seat crying hysterically. They were obviously terrorized by the whole ordeal.

Soon the police arrived, and Tom was taken to jail. His wife had to bail him out.

Was it worth it? Of course not!

Was it avoidable? Absolutely!

Ask yourself, "At what moment could the scenario have gone completely different?" Answer: at the moment of decision, when Tom made a choice to react in an angry and destructive way.

When Tom made the choice to throw his brain's executive function (the executive function or "frontal lobe" is the most developed cortex of the brain and is responsible for interpreting data, forming strategies, and making decisions) "out of the window," and chose to ignore any internal warning, he gave in to the urge to respond emotionally, out of fear, by striking back. This is precisely the moment at which "All Hell broke loose," producing a flood of electro-chemical responses that made the slippery slope of return to reason nearly impossible (of course the *Pons*, a portion of the brain responsible for managing fight and flight responses, could potentially need some strengthening in Tom's case as well).

As you can see from these illustrations, successful relating begins with the willingness and ability to choose well early on, as opposed to waiting for things to get out of hand.

As crude a weapon of the Cave man's club, the chemical barrage has been hurled against the fabric of life.

-Rachel Louise Carson

Session Recap of Barriers to Choosing Well

As we have just reviewed, in order to make good choices, you have to first ensure that your brain is free from "toxic" influencers, and has a healthy neuronal make-up from which to draw.

In the following, we will recap the toxic influencers that most often present barriers to making good decisions.

Destructive and Limiting Mind Tapes such as, "You will never amount to anything," or "You must do things our way," or "It is not okay for you to express your feelings."

These messages, often reinforced while a person is young and impressionable, become a physical part of his or her brain wiring. They affect virtually every area of that person's life—stripping confidence, and confining them to a life of listlessness, hopelessness, indecision, and despair.

Unprocessed Grief is being stuck in a phase of the grief cycle wherein resolution has never quite been achieved. In such cases, positive mind scaffolds (*scaffolds* are similar to clusters, in that, they represent a substantial or predominant networking of thoughts or an attitude) have never been established to resolve the pain of grief in a constructive and healthy way.

Traumatic Experiences & Painful Memories remain stored and bound-up within one's subconscious mind, leaving unprocessed incidence of trauma, emotional pain, disappointment, anger, and even rage. These influence a person's health and daily decisions to a far greater degree than may often be realized.

Our subconscious mind is incredibly powerful. It works much faster than our conscious mind, producing *billions* of actions per second. The conscious mind produces far less, *tens of thousands*, actions per second.

This being the case, the subconscious mind is in the business of accessing memories and the emotions attached to them every time we experience new input from our five senses. Upon attaching familiarity to the memories and emotions, the brain begins the process of interpretation.

Consistent with the phenomenon discussed in the section entitled, "Psychoemotional Drag," memories often "color" new experiences by reminding a person of old experiences, potentially releasing a host of displaced thoughts and feelings in their train (as discussed above—see on Norma's story).

Everything stored within your mind, virtually all memories, are a very real and physical part of *you*. You cannot hide them, or run from them, or pretend they do not exist. They will ultimately manifest in some way.

Negative thoughts, memories, and emotions are often the reason we make certain lifestyle decisions, influencing what we eat, say, and do. That is why unhealthy habits, such as, consuming too much sugar, sodas, tobacco, and even working, or working out too much, etc. often become ways of coping. These habits or addictions help us (superficially of course) cope with unresolved stress—as they provide temporary relief in response to toxic, energy draining loads on the brain.

Distorted Perceptions lead to distorted thinking. Many times we make poor, life-limiting decisions because we simply do not know any better. For example, the wiring of our brain interprets something as A, B, or C, while a more accurate interpretation, representing reality, can be found in X, Y, or Z.

Additionally, sometimes our own personal experience, or frame of reference, becomes our own worst enemy. We think something is true because we *thought* it to be so based on a limited perspective or within an entirely different context than would warrant the conclusions we have reached.

Toxic Influencers are around us everywhere. Negative news, television programs, billboard ads, adverse financial circumstances, and sometimes negative people can wreak havoc on our minds by the toxic ways in which they influence us.

I once read a sign over the exit of a gym listing the top ten strategies for success. What was listed as number one? "Avoid negative people!" I will likely never forget that sign.

We need eleven positive thoughts to balance one negative thought.
-Albert Einstein

Further Signs of a Toxic Mind Forest

Negative or distorted thinking; lack of energy, including fatigue and certain forms of depression; failure to follow through with commitments; impulsivity; mood swings; social withdrawal; addictive behavior; inappropriate or unwarranted anger (anger that is out of proportion to the event); unresolved sadness (crying for seemingly no reason); bouts with guilt; incessant "I should" or "I have to" statements; anxiety; panic attacks; phobias; obsessive compulsive behavior; a fear based or perfectionist mindset; codependence on someone or something to meet our needs; personal instability; sexual promiscuity; poor or underdeveloped judgment; self sabotaging behavior; hatred; victim mentality; unforgiveness and resentment; incessant lying; the need to convince others of "how great or accomplished I am"; frequent negative events or accidents; health problems and the like, all represent a toxic brain.

In place of these negative influencers, we must plant new, healthy seeds of positivity, possibility, and success. We must "clear the forest" of our mind, and plant seeds that are consistent with who we really are, so we can capture more of who we were created to become.

Recognizing the Common Roots of Failure: A Get Up! First Step

As we have seen thus far, there are many potential pitfalls that can drag a person down.

The good news remains that recognizing these pitfalls is the first step towards overcoming them.

Moving Forward

Entering into Sessions Three and Four, we will examine how the brain functions. It is important that we become more deeply acquainted with the underlying dynamics and processes involved in uprooting the common roots of failure. Because when the mystery of how our minds work is removed, the fear of the unknown loses its debilitating grip, and we become empowered and more skilled in its proper use.

Session Five will provide practical application of what you are learning, so that by following the exercises contained, you can knock out these common roots of failure and move forward towards becoming more of the person you were created to be—positive, effective, and more fully alive!

Session Three

Heart of the Matter

The mind is its own place, and in itself
Can make a Heaven or Hell.

–John Milton, Paradise Lost

Amazing Brain, How Sweet the Possibilities

Since your life is controlled in large part by your brain, it is essential that you spend some time becoming better acquainted with this amazing organ. That way you can begin orchestrating personal growth with maximum efficiency as you create your blueprint for life recovery and success.

Brain Interstate 101

The brain is a complex and highly sophisticated machine, arguably the most awesome of all human organs.

Its physical consistency is likened to that of custard. In fact, a living brain is so soft that it can be cut with a butter knife. "Don't try this at home!"

The brain weighs approximately three pounds.

Brain neurons are typically the oldest cells in your body.

"A newborn brain contains something on the order of 100,000,000,000—that's 100 billion—nerve cells. That is most of the neurons a brain will ever have" (Schwartz & Begley, 2002).

Did you know that brain neurons happen to be the longest cells in your body? In some cases, a neuron may be up to three (3) feet long. Perhaps that's why people say, "A little knowledge goes a long way!" (Jaguar Educational, 2010).

"The brain's various parts and its nerve cells are connected by nearly 1 million miles of nerve fibers. The human brain has the largest area of uncommitted cortex (with no specific function identified so far) of any species on earth. This gives humans extraordinary flexibility for learning" (Jensen, 2005).

The brain is powerful. The fact is, however, we only tap into approximately 2-3% of its raw power.

The brain is dynamic. It is ever adapting in response to new stimuli introduced daily through the five senses.

The pioneering neurophysiologist Sir Charles Sherrington, in an oft' quoted passage, describes the brain this way: "It is as if the Milky Way entered upon some cosmic dance. Swiftly, the brain becomes an enchanted loom where millions of flashing shuttles weave a dissolving pattern, always a meaningful pattern though never an abiding one; a shifting harmony of subpatterns" (Restak, 1994).

Visual organization studies were among the first to provide evidence to neuroscientists that there seem to be parts of the brain, "modules", that perform functions quite independent of other "modules" (Restak, 1994).

Nevertheless, the brain is highly integrated. Brain structures often compete and cooperate. Recognizing the systemic (functions as an interrelated organ) nature of the brain helps us better understand the compounding synergistic dynamics sparked upon impact of one area of the brains function, and conversely, the obstacles introduced when a particular area of our brain is not functioning properly or is compromised in some way (Jenson, 2005).

The relationship does not end here.

Research studies show that a person's brain function is closely associated with their physical health.

The brain consumes more of the body's energy supply than any other organ. In fact, approximately 20% of the body's blood and oxygen supply are utilized by the brain. It provides enough energy to light a light bulb! (Jaguar Educational, 2010).

Indeed, the brain is an amazing organ!

Understanding the internal dynamics of brain change serves as an important prelude to applying the New Mind Synergy (NMS = CG2) formula for success strategies as outlined in the following sessions.

The Plastic Brain: Privilege and Responsibility

Since the brain is adaptable and changeable, the term "plastic" is a fitting descriptor—the understanding of which represents both a *privilege* and a *responsibility*. It represents a privilege because it invites an individual to strive to become all that God has created him or her to be, regardless of the past. It means the opportunity for a person to overhaul his or her life and develop into his or her unique gift to the world. It represents a responsibility because the potential for negative development exists as well—what is often called, in the field of neuroscience, the "paradox of plasticity."

The paradox of plasticity recognizes that just as positive changes in your brain can be made through positive thoughts, desires, choices, and actions, so negative changes can be established just the same.

You do well to daily consider the results of your choices on the development of your brain—especially since every habit, thought, and experience becomes a very real, physical part of *you*.

What Do You Truly Want?

Have you asked yourself this question, "What is it that I *truly* desire for my life?" Do you want an increased sense of personal happiness; a new career; increased earnings; a better quality of life; a more positive attitude; increased wisdom, knowledge, or learning potential; better time and money management skills; freedom from an addiction; increased personal discipline; more joy, peace, energy, or confidence; improved connections with others; or the discipline to consistently abide by the values that you hold most dear? The good news is that truly anything you desire, and want seriously enough, is possible to you.

The *choice* is yours.

In order to capitalize on the power of thoughts, and use our brains for maximum benefit, we must both *desire* and *choose* to do so.

Desire Comes from Within

The economies of desire and choice are the only accounts to which another person cannot make a deposit on your behalf. While I or someone else can help fan the flames of desire and encourage you to make healthy choices, ultimately desire and the freedom to choose are yours and yours alone.

Good stewardship of both desire and freedom of choice demand personal responsibility just as equally as they represent pathways of opportunity.

Imagine being locked into your current condition, fate sealed by the shackles of adverse genetic or environmental conditions. At least, with choices there is hope for change and a brighter tomorrow.

Which leads to the following question: "Have you ever pondered why it is that some people choose to seek the very best for their lives, while others settle for far less?"

You Only Live Once!

Darren Hardy, publisher and Editorial Director of *Seeds of Success* Magazine, in a September 7, 2010 newsletter message entitled, "The Greatest Goal and Purpose in Life", writes, "Unfortunately, many people don't dare to dream about what they can achieve. They lock their greatness away, afraid of their own vast potential. Instead of stepping out of their comfort zone, they deny life's possibilities and choose to live safe . . . and small. It is said that the greatest waste in the world is the difference between what we are and what we are capable of becoming."

If this sounds familiar, then I urge you to stop living in a haphazard manner. Take your life "by the horns," and begin living with greater intentionality. After all, life is not a spectator event!

And just so that you remain balanced in your perspective on this matter, it is important to remember that many people would choose change (they have a heart to do so), and latch onto greater opportunity, if they were just shown how. That is the very reason for which this book is written, to help show the way.

Oftentimes, when I see a person who appears to be living below his or her potential, or suffering the consequences of self-limiting or poor life choices, I endeavor to maintain a balanced perspective regarding the reality of personal responsibility on one hand, and that person's potentially deep inner desire for change on the other.

On Judging Others

Ultimately, it is far better to love and embrace people for who they are. I encourage you not to use the fact that they *can* change and *do* have a choice as an excuse to form a moralistic position against them.

Morality is good. However, being moralistic is something quite different. A moralist is someone who wears morality on his or her sleeve, similar to a badge of honor.

Oftentimes, I find that moralistic people are guilty of some of the more severe violations against others. In fact, their gravitation toward adopting a moralistic posture seems more an attempt to compensate for personal insecurity, than anything else.

People are the way they are for many reasons. And in the end, who are we to judge?

Sometimes it can take years of committed effort and focused intervention to reverse certain negative tendencies and to form more constructive and enduring characteristics. It all depends on the person and the kinds of change under consideration in any given circumstance. In almost every case, change occurs because a loving friend, coach, mentor, or family member came along side to help.

Our job is simply to love people and endeavor to be a catalyst for change. We can help by rolling up our sleeves, getting involved, and then patiently showing others the way.

As one of my mentors and dear friends, Dr. Ian Chand (for years the Clinical Director of Loma Linda University's Department of Counseling and Family Sciences, and truly one of the most gracious men that I have ever been privileged to know), taught me years ago, "You cannot be somebody's judge and friend at the same time."

Particularly for those in positions of authority, when it's a tough call, but wherein a decision must be made to either discipline a person for their actions, or show grace—in close situations if you are going to error at all—it is better to error on the side of mercy, rather than judgment."

-Dr. Jack Blanco

Heart of the Matter—choice!

What is mind? No matter. What is matter? Never mind.

-T.H. Key

The choices we make ultimately stem from deep within the heart—the mind, soul, and spirit of a man or woman—and therefore, are determined at a level that cannot be studied under a microscope. This being the case, mind does not matter; it does not present itself as actual physical matter. So then what exactly does it mean when we talk about the heart, and whether or not it really *matters*?

Despite T.H. Keys' clever play on words in the epigraph cited above, this is a very important question that will be answered as follows: The term "heart" is often used synonymously with "mind," "soul," and "spirit," and yes it matters a great deal, because it is essentially *you*—character, and to some degree, personality.

For as a man thinks in his heart, so is he.

-Proverbs 23:7

Your mind, will, and emotions form the components of what we often refer to as soul. Soul also happens to be where personal choice is seated, acting in concert with your spirit.

The spirit and soul (mind) of a person, though unique entities, are untraceably linked and are often loosely referred to synonymously.

The actual physical make-up of the brain (its biology, including genetics and environmental shaping) works in concert with spirit and soul to both shape and express the unique "flavor" of the individual personality.

Going back a few paragraphs, the words "and to some degree, personality" have been carefully chosen for a particular reason. That is because while spirit does indeed represent the essence of your personality, we must remember that whatever the mind, soul, spirit, or heart of a man or woman seeks to express must first "filter through" the physical structure of the brain. Put simply, a healthy brain equates with a clear representation of the personality, while an unhealthy brain equates with an unclear or distorted representation of the personality.

This remains the case until we learn to transcend whatever cognitive negativity exists within the physical matter of our brain—negativity that is established through genetics, as well as shaped by our environment.

The question is whether such a technique can really make a man good. Greatness comes from within. . . . Goodness is something chosen. When a man cannot choose he ceases to be a man.

-Anthony Burgess, A Clockwork Orange

As one might imagine, for centuries debates have often focused on questions regarding the nature of the mind, and more specifically, its origin. For instance, if the mind and individuality, as materialists suggest, is merely an expression of, and limited to, the physical matter that houses and supports it, then there really is no such thing as free will. This perspective is what is often referred to as "determinism." Determinists believe that a person's destiny is predetermined by genetics and environmental shaping, independent of a personal choice variable.

Jeffrey M. Schwartz, M.D., and Sharon Begley (2002-2003), frame it this way:

...neuroscience has linked genetic mechanisms to neuronal circuits coursing with a multiplicity of neurotransmitters to argue that the brain is a machine whose behavior is predestined, or at least determined, in such a way as seemingly to leave no room for the will. It is not merely that the will is not free, in the modern scientific view; not merely that it is constrained, a captive of material forces. It is, more radically, that the will, a manifestation of mind, does not even exist, because a mind independent of brain does not exist.

On the other hand, an individual who believes that we are more than physical matter and that soul and spirit represent the very essence of life, relegating the material body to a mere structure, vehicle, or mode of expression, arrives at a vastly different conclusion.

Both premises embrace the reality of brain change and seek to explain it, albeit with differing conclusions as to ultimate origins. The former denies the concept of underlying responsibility associated with free will, while the latter embraces it—blazing an exciting trail of increased potentiality with implications for this life, and hope for one to come.

Above all else, guard your heart, for it is the wellspring of life.
-Jesus Christ

Epigenetics, The Science of Choice

Now let's go a bit deeper by examining the specific brain mechanisms associated with choice.

In biology, epigenetics is the study of inherited changes in phenotype, i.e., appearance or gene expression caused by mechanisms other than changes in the underlying DNA sequence. Hence the name "epi-" (Greek for "over" or "above") genetics.

Robin Holiday, Ph.D., a molecular biologist, defined epigenetics as "the study of the mechanisms of temporal and spatial control of gene activity during the development of complex organisms. Thus, epigenetics can be used to describe anything other than DNA sequence that influences the development of an organism" (Holiday, 1990).

Psychologist Erik Erikson used the term in his theory of psychosocial development. In Erikson's view, individuals go through several developmental stages, the transition through each being marked by a crisis.

According to Erickson, although the stages are predetermined by genetics, the way in which a person resolves the crisis is not; by comparison of the epigenetic theory of cell differentiation, the process was said to be epigenetic.

The study of epigenetics ultimately refers to the ways in which our environment, and our responses to it, via the choices that we make, impact our development, and hence, our lives and those of our offspring. This dynamic phenomenon ultimately links back to our earlier discussion about neuroplasticity and the ability of the brain to change, adapt, and develop according to how we choose to program and nurture it.

Neurogenesis

Studies in neurogenesis, which is the creation of new brain neurons, push the envelope even further beyond epigenetics (changes at the molecular level of an *already existing neuron*). Scientists such as Fred Gage; together with colleagues at the Salk Institute in La Jolla; Elizabeth Gould of Princeton University; and Peter Eriksson of Goteborg, Sweden have discovered the actual *creation of new neurons* (Schwart and Begley, 2002).

Their studies suggest that the possibilities for neuroplasticity are greater than even diehard neuroplasticity proponents had previously thought, and that the brain may not be limited to working with already existing neurons, but may actually add fresh neurons into the mix. "The neural electrician is not restricted to working with existing wiring, we now know: he can run whole new cables through the brain" (Schwartz & Begley, 2002).

All of this lends further proof to the premise that we *can* alter our destiny, as well as that of our offspring. We are not bound by predetermined genetics. We can make the choice to excel.

Choose Life

A powerful scripture verse relaying the power of choice is found in Deuteronomy 30:19, "I have set before you life and death, the blessing and the curse. So choose life in order that you may live, you and your descendants" (Deuteronomy 30:19).

It is truly amazing, and certainly humbling, that we can alter the destiny of not only ourselves, but of our offspring, for *several generations to come!*

What choices will YOU make?

SESSION FOUR

DESTROYING ROOTS OF FAILURE

The brain is the violin and the soul is the violinist. They both need to work together in order to make beautiful music.

-Father Charles Ara, Catholic Priest

The Brain's Seek-and-Destroy Mechanism

As alluded to earlier, the brain has a built-in "seek-and-destroy" mechanism (SDM) that operates to both manage and destroy "toxic" and negative thoughts. Since thoughts grow branches and multiply in kind, they eventually become grouped or clustered together. A conglomeration of negative thoughts adversely influences ones attitude, behavior, and emotions.

According to Dr. Leaf, " . . . we have billions of existing thought clusters with their emotions attached giving their specific attitude [or] 'flavor' . . . and every type of emotion has one of only two roots – love or fear. Love and fear are the root emotions, and all other emotions grow from these." She continues, "Science is showing us there is a massive 'unlearning' of negative toxic thoughts when we operate in love. The brain releases a chemical called oxytocin, which literally melts away the negative toxic thought clusters so that rewiring of new non-toxic circuits can happen. This chemical also flows when we trust and bond and reach out to others. Love literally wipes out fear!" (Leaf, 2009).

Consider this for a moment: if everything in your life can be boiled down to either love or fear, would this not help simplify matters a great deal?

If you came to understand your toxic thoughts as stemming from fear, would this not present an opportunity to grasp a better handle on your life and what may be driving you?

Conversely, since love—as manifest by nurturing oneself and others, showing patience and kindness, making healthy life decisions, or offering a gentle touch to someone in need—actually has a healthy effect on your brain, doesn't this sound like an attractive way to restructure your thinking and begin to transform your life?

Besides oxytocin, other electro-chemicals, such as dopamine, give us a positive "charge" whenever we anticipate something favorable or become excited in a positive way. These electro-chemicals have a positive impact on our thoughts, motivation levels, and mental make-up.

Additionally, serotonin and a few other chemicals are essential components of a loving, positive, stable, and optimally functioning brain.

It is amazing to think that electro-chemicals, activated by making healthy and loving choices, can trigger a seek-and-destroy mechanism that literally melts away negative thoughts!

The brain's seek-and-destroy mechanism is only effective to the degree that it has enough healthy neuronal trees and branches to accomplish the mission efficiently. This is primarily because if the negativity is intense enough, i.e., an overabundance of unhealthy neuronal branches and trees when compared with that of healthy neuronal branches and trees, then the healthy neurons that *do* exist are over taxed and electro-chemically become imbalanced, resulting in decreased efficiency, and therefore, diminished effectiveness of SDM. The result of this is a depletion of available resources and energy that might otherwise be used for other important functions, resulting in depression, fatigue, diminished concentration, and increased stress.

This is precisely why people with an unhealthy mindset are tired a good part of the time. It is a lot of work to try and manage toxic trees and branches.

Socially speaking, people with depleted cognitive function often report a decrease in personal confidence, exuberance, memory, spontaneity and present mindedness—often failing to remain "in the moment." That is because resources are being diverted to manage negative thoughts and are creating disorder to the electro-chemical reactions within the brain, resulting in confusion and a restriction of freedom to more fully engage in a socially meaningful way.

Similar dynamics hold true for physical health, academic, professional, and various personal pursuits; resulting in a decreased quality of performance, and therefore, a decreased quality of life.

Destroying Toxic Mind Trees & Planting Healthy Mind Trees

Since each nerve cell in your brain looks like a tree with a central cell body and branches, a leading researcher at the University of California at Berkeley, Marion Diamond, together with an award winning science writer, Janet Hopson, refer to neuronal branches as "the magic trees of the mind" (1999).

Dr. Leaf (2010), in an interview with marketing expert, entrepreneur, and success coach, Ali Brown, further enhanced my understanding of the trees of the mind by offering a colorful analogy. She referred to healthy trees of the mind as "green trees," and toxic trees of the mind as "black trees." Dr. Leaf explained that on a microscopic level, neuronal trees and branches have a unique appearance similar to what we might see, for example, in a forest, when comparing a healthy, vibrant, green tree to that of a tree that is dying. She teaches that green trees represent love, while black trees represent fear, and that, "We are wired to build green trees. . . . We are wired for love. . . . The black trees are hijackers. They are not supposed to be there. This is not according to God's order and design." She further contends that issues such as forgiveness and unforgiveness build physically into the brain and that we can choose to build in a positive or a negative direction. Furthermore, says Leaf, "'I can't' is not neutral. . . . It's a decision. . . . Forgiveness [via built-in brain processes, mechanisms, and chemicals] destroys . . . melts away into gas . . . black trees," and fosters the development of green trees. What is the result of this dynamic process? A new green tree thought strand begins to enhance one's ability to operate from love, as opposed to fear.

I have referred to Dr. Leaf's illustration of the green and black trees in work with my clients and in a few workshops where I have presented on the topic of cleansing toxic thoughts. The audience catches the concept almost immediately. They absolutely love it!

Should my clients find themselves becoming stuck and feeling negative, overly stressed, or defeated, I often remind them to "Keep planting that forest of green trees." Almost without fail, I will get a call or text some time later saying, "Thank you! What you said really helped. Things got better after you reminded me to keep planting green trees."

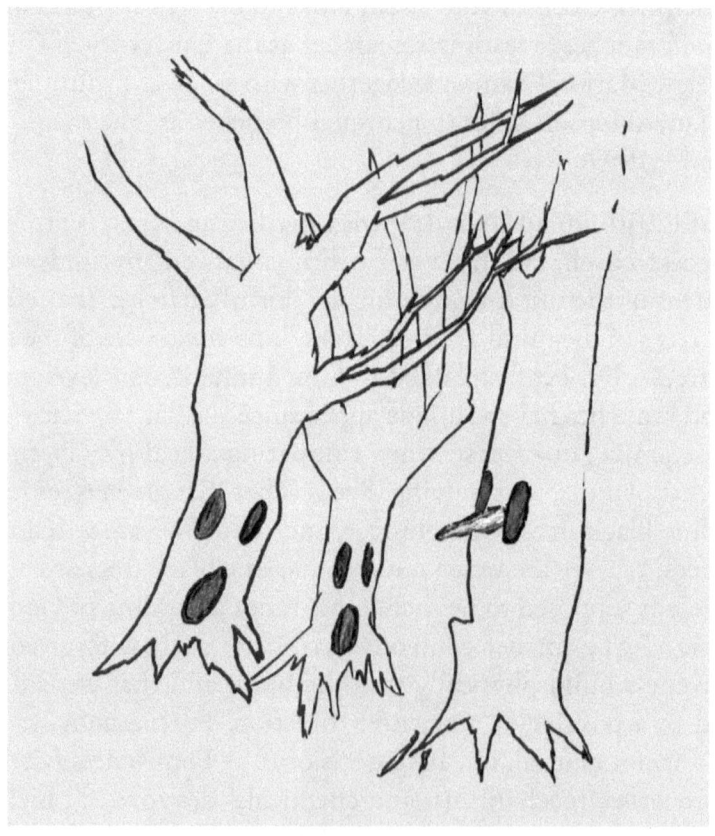

"Spooky" "black" trees of fear

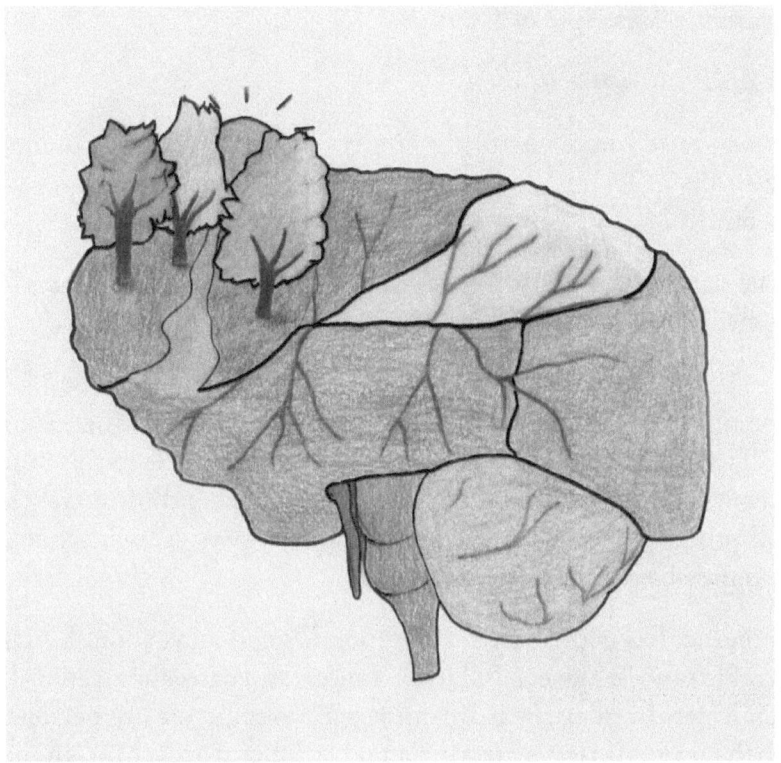

Healthy "green" trees of the mind, representing love.

A Window of Opportunity

Something that I learned while training in hypnotherapy and in research on the subject of cognitive change processes is the fact that the moment a memory moves from the unconscious to the conscious mind, it can be changed. This is where a window of opportunity exists for reconsolidation to take place as new proteins are formed following retrieval (Tronson & Taylor, 2007) and (Nader, Schafe, & Doux, 2000).

The goal of therapy is to help a client recall troubling and unresolved memories, and then to reorganize such memories in a healthier way. While there are a variety of techniques to accomplish this, we will review many of the most essential strategies (some you can practice yourself) throughout the remainder of Part One.

A Dramatic Example of Change

Meet Anil

Anil was raised in a nurturing family. He described his parents and older sisters as loving, and related feeling fortunate to be from such a good family.

For the past several years, he has attended a private college located close to home. His ultimate goal has been to work his way through the ranks and eventually be a public school administrator.

Unfortunately, and unbeknownst to his parents at the time, Anil was sexually abused as a child by a trusted family friend. He recalls how this occurrence stripped him of personal confidence, and ultimately led to sexual promiscuity that started his freshman year of high school, and has progressively gotten worse.

His conduct has contributed to compounding doubts about his chosen career. He says, "How can I plan on a successful career as an educational leader, a person of trust, if I cannot get a handle on my personal life and behavior?" This was creating a real conflict within him. In fact, he even changed majors believing that he would never "have it together" enough to be a leader. The conflict and indecision this created was grueling for Anil!

The shame of the abuse incident lay dormant within Anil for many years and was stripping him of personal confidence and his ability to fully express his leadership gifts. He reported often being tired and irritable.

Anil's energy was consumed by trying to suppress and manage the shame of the abuse that he had encountered, and the irrational belief that he was somehow responsible for what had occurred.

After numerous prior attempts at psychotherapy, he came to me for help. We attacked Anil's issue by utilizing the principles of the New Mind Synergy formula.

First, we got a good handle on the extent and nature of the abuse. Then, in a relaxed setting, I suggested that Anil recall the event as clearly and specifically as possible. Upon being ready, Anil invited his abuser into the room (in imagination) and confronted him, expressing the pain he was forced to endure as a result of the acts that were committed against him (this is a very important step in the grief process).

Over the course of a few sessions, Anil was able to fully process the incident and reorganize it. Since Anil was able to express his feelings of hurt towards his abuser, then reframe and lay strength to it, he was able to reorganize it in a healthier way.

Ultimately, Anil was able to forgive his perpetrator. This further contributed towards the development of a healthy new brain cluster, based on self-acceptance, forgiveness, and love; as opposed to shame, resentment, and fear.

This exercise had a powerful affect on Anil's life.

For several weeks his countenance maintained an incessant glow, as though the weight of the world was lifted from his shoulders. By making the choice to do the hard work required to be healthy, Anil triumphed over that which held him hostage for so long.

This victory allowed us to move into a goals-oriented coaching component where he reaffirmed his academic and professional goals and was able to rediscover his life's possibility and potential. He is now free to exercise his gift of leadership and service to others.

The Perils of an Empty Love Bank

In our Western culture today, there are many who do not have the intimacy they desire built into their lives, resulting in loneliness and isolation. Failure to form intimacy is among the primary culprits responsible for addictive behavior (and psychological maladjustment). We often medicate ourselves to take the place of the bonds that should exist by virtue of family and friendship connections.

In a cultural climate wherein so many of us are scrambling just to survive, busyness often trumps relationship. When this occurs, the human heart suffers from an intimacy void.

A Shot of Intimacy

I recently heard a woman describe being at a family reunion for the first time in years. She recalled, "The experience with family was so full, so rich, that it filled my heart to overflowing."

The last thing on a person's mind at such an event is to resort to an addiction (although, some families are capable of triggering an addiction!), because his or her love bank is so full. As a result, the individual feels "high" from oxytocin, flowing freely like whiskey at a Saturday night bonfire on 2nd and Main!

Unfortunately, the following day, week, or month ushers in that all-too-familiar return to normal life, where the day-to-day feeling of isolation re-emerges—the void so prevalent in addictive behavior.

It may not surprise you to learn that the woman then begged this question: "Have you ever noticed that family reunions just don't seem to last long enough?"

Do You Feel A Loss?

Perhaps you feel a loss because you do not have a mother, father, brother, sister, grandparent, or extended family member with whom you can connect. Lonely and set adrift, you grieve, because you think, "Man, if I just had a family, my pain would go away!"

Maybe you can even track the many ways in which this unmet need has demanded a hefty toll from your life.

Healthy Ways to Build Intimacy

A few possible ways to build intimacy into your life are to create or join a small group, establish a community of friends, fellowship at church, or strengthen ties with family members by making a focused and determined effort to reconnect. Don't wait for others to initiate contact. Building intimacy sometimes requires that you be the one who makes the first move. You might even be surprised to learn that those individuals with whom you desire more contact are hoping for the same. They just don't know how to reach out.

Maintaining Intimacy

We need to have the mentality of bridge-builders if we are to maintain intimacy. We cannot focus on the imperfections of others, or retreat when they do not respond to us as we think they should. It is hard to form intimate community and be thin-skinned at the same time.

Let's face it. Humans are imperfect. Given enough time, or the right circumstances, we are all capable of letting others, even those we love and adore, down. However, a bridge-builder makes a conscious decision to focus on the good in others, and as a result, maintains more friendships. Now get out there and embrace the good in others!

The Human Element

Ultimately, regardless of the program or technique that a therapist may use to foster change in a client's life, the element of human interaction is what ultimately provides the healing balm. That is why I am such a big proponent of individual therapy, one-to-one mentoring, and small group work.

In our Western culture, as I mentioned in Session Two, Perfectionists, we have a tendency to believe that we cannot allow others to know us for who we *really* are. We hide behind a façade of who we think we are *supposed* to be. After all, we think we must be strong and "have it all together." If this sounds familiar, I urge you to join a small group wherein you can share your humanness—pain, struggles, disappointments, and failures—in a safe atmosphere of love and acceptance. For some, this is an incredibly freeing and important step towards experiencing true intimacy, and the psychological well-being that only human connection can give.

Session Four Summary

Albert Einstein is quoted as having said, "Amidst difficulty lies opportunity." Decide at this moment to seize opportunity by taking personal responsibility for growing through your present difficulties. Chances are that many of your difficulties are self-created: the fruit of a toxic mind. Begin by establishing a healthy state of mind.

Like Anil, get with a therapist and do the work required to begin reprogramming the toxic thoughts that have held you captive, and which contribute to fear, confusion, and self sabotage. Your new mentality will forge a pathway to greater mental clarity, unbridled personal growth, and life success.

Moving Forward

As we move through the remainder of Part One, start thinking about how the information presented thus far in Sessions One, Two, Three, and Four can be applied through the techniques that will now be introduced in Session Five.

Remember, Part One, *cognition*, will ultimately pair with Part Two, *goals*, creating a synergistic explosion of healthy trees of the mind *and* a more focused, positive, and powerful life direction.

GROWING A HEALTHY
MIND FOREST

A prudent man gives thought to his steps.
-Proverbs 14:15

Arriving now at Session Five, you have already been introduced to the concept of brain plasticity, i.e., brain changeability, adaptability, and modifiability—the "abilities"—pleasure to meet you! Also, you have explored the concept of personal growth and transformation via the New Mind Synergy formula for success (NMS=CG2). And by this point in your reading, maybe you've even identified the roots of failure responsible for sabotaging your personal progress for all of these years. Remember, the power of choice, i.e., the ability to alter your life's destiny, and that of your offspring for generations to come—by the choices you make from this point forward—is yours for the taking. With this understanding, you are now ready to focus on techniques that will help you apply what you have learned thus far.

What Makes New Mind Synergy So Unique?

Many goals programs never address the underlying reasons *why* failure keeps occurring in a person's life.

I made the decision to include the common roots of failure (Session Two) as a prelude to the goals portion of the book because I have come to understand the absolute necessity of healthy cognition as a prelude to success, and because I realize that fear of the unknown (the "mysteries of the mind") blinds our ability to see that change is indeed possible. We are often afraid of the unfamiliar, leaving the fog of confusion to maintain its stifling grip.

It is often said, "Knowledge is power." This is especially true when dealing with the underlying dynamics that influence our thoughts, feelings, and behavior. By being armed with knowledge about the mind we can apply effective strategies and techniques as we prepare to Get Up!, fight the battle, and *win*.

Cognitive Programming Techniques

Dr. Daniel Amen, clinical neuroscientist, psychiatrist, and medical director of the Amen Clinics asserts that "Optimizing your life has a positive impact on brain function. As brain function impacts behavior, so too does behavior impact the brain. There is scientific evidence that living a positive, spiritual life, improves brain function. As with computers, hardware problems in the brain can be helped by special programming techniques [exercises] or software" (2002).

In the following, we will review a few of the very best techniques (some of which can be practiced at home, while others are best utilized via the assistance of a trained mental health professional).

Magic Pill

The "Magic Pill" technique is something I learned in graduate school. This intervention asks the question, "If you could take a magic pill that would resolve all of your life's troubles and worries, and then wake to find that somehow everything is brand new, what would be different?" This technique is similar to the Major Definite Purpose (MDP) question that will be introduced in Part Two (Tracy, 2003).

I really like this exercise because it provides an organized way to get in touch with what is weighing on a person, what is holding him or her back, and essentially, where it hurts.

Any time we have an opportunity to bring our cares, worries, and concerns from deep within, where we can better express, understand, and organize them, we have won half of the battle. In my work over the years, I have discovered that people sometimes feel anxious and depressed, but haven't the faintest clue why.

Inviting disappointments, fears, and painful memories to emerge from the unconscious and subconscious minds to the conscious mind provides a person with an opportunity to confront and process cognitive toxicity in an intentional, healthy, and solution-oriented way.

When you ask yourself the "magic pill" question, you may be surprised at what surfaces.

You will want to write down your responses on a sheet of paper. By writing things down, not only are you able to actually see what is ailing you, but you then have the added benefit of releasing it from your mind, and getting it out onto paper. This is a tremendously freeing exercise.

When completing this exercise, you do not need to write a book. Instead, try using succinct sentences that will serve as a list, as these can be expressed in further detail when you create your blueprint for life success (Session Ten). Additionally, rather than focusing solely on negative issues, you will want to build into your life enough positivity to propel you over the obstacles that you face presently. Remember, it is always better to deal with negativity by reframing the situation and finding a positive solution (for more on this, refer ahead to Session Eleven).

Any time a person wants to stop an unhealthy habit or behavior, it is best to implement a healthy alternative that he or she can enjoy instead. I always encourage my clients to focus less on running *from*, and more on running *to*, something better. Allow me to further illustrate by the following question: if you are driving your car and wish to make it from point A to point B without an accident, should you focus on the ditch alongside the road, or on the road itself? The answer is obvious.

A similar principle applies to fear-based tactics. Fear does not typically enhance true change. Instead, positivity, and enthusiasm for what is good, does.

Later on, while creating your blueprint for life success, you will synergistically discover solutions to some of the more perplexing issues facing you at the present time. Mountains that seem to loom like giants before you will begin to dissolve as a result of the positivity being built into your life.

One Page Miracle for the Soul

A technique shared by Dr. Amen in his book *Healing the Hardware of the Soul* is the One Page Miracle for the Soul.

At the top of a clean sheet of paper, write, "What do I really want?" *and* "What am I doing to make it happen?"

Then, in four separate categories write the following:

Relationships
Spouse/Lover:
Children:
Friends:
Family:

Work/Finances
Current/Short Term:
Future:
Finances:

Self
Physical:
Emotional:
Interests:

Soul
Spirit:
Relationship with God:
Character / Personality:

According to Dr. Amen, this exercise "enhances prefrontal cortex functioning by helping you focus on eternal values for your life . . . and allows . . . [you] . . . to see beyond the moment and plan for the future, enhancing decision-making ability and judgment; which assists . . . [you] . . . in avoiding impulsive, destructive, and potentially life-altering decisions." This exercise helps you feel focused, organized, and hopeful more quickly than almost any other exercise of which I am aware.

You may want to start by first writing, on a separate sheet of paper, your values for each category, e.g., Personal Wisdom; Wealth; Fulfilling Relationships; Fame; Personal Accomplishments; Leaving a Legacy; Honesty and Integrity; Faith in Yourself; Faith in a Higher Power; and How You Appear to Others. Then write down what you are doing right now to accomplish these important items that you've placed on your list (Amen, 2002).

I recall some seven years ago when I personally completed this exercise. It had a powerful impact on my life. I still carry the paper from that original exercise. It is laminated and remains in my wallet at all times. I review it daily before leaving the house, then again at night before going to bed, and sometimes even when waiting for something or someone while I'm out running errands.

. . . whatever is true, whatever is noble, whatever is right, whatever is pure, whatever is lovely, whatever is admirable—if anything is excellent or praiseworthy—think about such things.

-Philippians 4:8-9

Challenging Distorted Thoughts and Beliefs

This is a simple, easy to use technique. It simply means that you become more aware of your thoughts, rather than just passively receiving whatever comes to mind. This way you can better decide if your thoughts are true or not, and you can either accept or reject them based on reality, and not on distorted thinking. For example, if while completing this exercise a thought emerges that is untrue, than it can be rejected immediately. In its place you might say, "I reject this A, B, C thought, and instead, I accept X, Y, and Z as true."

A person can really have fun and play with this exercise a bit in order to further reinforce positivity. It's great when you get to the point where you can actually play with or chuckle at the negative thoughts!

This exercise is further enhanced when an individual is also a participant in either personal cognitive therapy or a cognitive therapy process group. A good cognitive therapist or savvy group setting often promotes valuable feedback which enables a person to better analyze his or her thoughts and beliefs.

We are disturbed not by things, but by the views we take of things.
-Epictetus, *The Encheiridion*

ANTS

The term ANT is an acronym for Automatic Negative Thoughts. These are thoughts that just appear seemingly from out of nowhere and seek to pervade a person's thoughts. They come in a variety of forms, are invasive, and really know how to "eat your lunch" if you let them!

They include:

Blaming - and failing to take personal responsibility.

Over-generalizing - such as "always" and "never" thinking.

Mind Reading - assuming that someone is thinking the worst about you, or must be upset, angry, or disappointed because he or she failed to greet, acknowledge, or react to you in a way you think they should.

Fortune Telling - assuming things will work out for the worst.

Disproportionate Self-Blame - criticizing and blaming oneself for even the slightest imperfection or infraction.

Thinking with Your Feelings - we alluded to this in the story about Tom, Session Two. From his example we understand why emotive thinking can be particularly destructive. Additionally, sometimes dating couples cannot separate their feelings from their decisions long enough to make healthy life choices. Been there! Done that!

Automatic Negative Thought Stopping is the remedy for negative, intrusive, or overly emotion-laden thoughts. ANTS exercises can easily be done at home and are to be practiced daily by those individuals serious about gaining control over the nature of their thoughts.

Every time a negative thought appears or you feel yourself heading down the slippery slope of negativity, simply stop the thought, switch your thinking to something more positive, and counteract the negativity with the truth of the matter.

For instance, ladies suppose you are driving along in your car and you see a billboard with a picture of a scantily clad, attractive woman, appearing to have all the guys at her fingertips. Your mind could potentially think, "I will never be that beautiful. I will never be able to attract a man. I am destined to a life of T.V. dinners, aloneness, and depression." Then, as if your thoughts were not already bad enough, your mind switches to recount all the failures you have ever experienced, and you find your mood spiraling DOWN, down, *down*. "Haagen-Dazs anyone?" This represents a bad case of ANT invasion.

In response, you can open up a can of "Whoop ANT Repellant!"—hopefully, immediately upon the initial thought entering your mind—by saying to yourself, "I am beautiful just the way I am. God made me unique and special for just the right guy. Besides, I am in control of my body, and if I choose to enhance my appearance in some way, I can and I will. I am capable of obtaining whatever it is I truly want. I will be successful." A sense of excitement will kick-in as you begin to plot just exactly how you are going to go about achieving your objectives for success.

This is far better than the alternative and more accurately represents the truth. Wouldn't you agree?

My clients who struggle with negative thoughts are often asked to create a list of personal strengths identifying five, ten, or fifteen personal attributes that they will review on a daily basis. This way, their ANT repellant is always on-the-ready.

I have had some clients over the years who have confessed, "I cannot think of anything good about myself." Together, we have no problem finding plenty of good things to add to their list.

Besides, even if they do not believe the truth about themselves, the subconscious mind does not discriminate between truth and non-truth, but simply logs input, stores it as true, and voila—a new healthy mind branch can still be formed.

There is nothing either good or bad, but thinking makes it so.
-William Shakespeare, *Hamlet*

Positive Affirmations

Positive affirmations are powerful. This is a quick, daily routine that works wonders in terms of developing a healthy mind forest and building personal confidence.

I make the habit of reading a list of positive affirmations every morning before I leave for work as part of my daily routine, and then again each night before bed.

A positive affirmations list is simply a list of five, ten, or fifteen positive things about yourself that you can say (out loud whenever possible) on a routine basis to send a positive message to your subconscious mind.

We all have mornings that we wake-up and something is weighing us down. We feel tired or something particularly negative greets us before the morning coffee even has a chance to brew!

I recall having such a morning a while back. I was wrestling with all the demands of the day and my mind was tempted to rehearse those areas where things may not yet be exactly as I would have them to be, *yet*.

Then I pulled out my positive affirmations, together with my goals and daily priority list, and reviewed them as I was getting ready to head to the office. Within minutes, my attitude shifted and I left the house that morning feeling confident and filled with possibility, as if standing in direct defiance of anything that would even dare to get in my way.

Since positive affirmations build healthy tree branches in the forest of the mind, they are a great gift-releaser. Every time we affirm a positive attribute in ourselves, our unique ability is further strengthened. This is fantastic, as it puts us in touch with our personal gifts and brings them top of mind where we can more readily position ourselves to operate from a place of strength, as opposed to operating from a position of weakness or personal vulnerability.

I am currently working with a client who is constantly reminded of his personal inadequacies every time he reports to work. Although he tries to ignore the well positioned jabs of criticism by his peers, eventually the tension builds to the point that he verbally explodes.

I told him, *"It is not enough to simply ignore the jabs, but you must build the positive scaffolds of your mind by rehearsing the truth about yourself so intensively and with such determination (through positive affirmations) that your gifts and the truth about yourself are top of mind at all times. In this way, you will not merely ignore the jabs, but will also be equipped to better evaluate them.*

By maintaining a powerful force of truth and positive energy in your mind, you will more readily identify the negativity for what it is, and therefore, become empowered to respond in a constructive way.

As you become increasingly capable of more accurately discerning between destructive criticism and constructive peer feedback, you become better able to learn and grow into your role as a professional.

As knowledge builds upon knowledge, your gifts and creative genius will emerge stronger unto automaticity [when we master something so well that we can do it as second nature—automatically], your confidence will grow, and you will stop second guessing your performance."

Both professionally and personally, we are not meant to come from a position of weakness (such as when we second guess ourselves), but are meant to operate increasingly from a position of strength.

Build positive affirmations into your daily routine. You will be amazed at the difference it makes!

I would rather go a morning without breakfast, than a morning without positive affirmations.
-Unknown

Deep Breathing Exercises, Meditation, Self Hypnosis and Journaling

Deep breathing has a profound effect on an individual's brain energy by bringing oxygen from the atmosphere and into the lungs. It has a relaxing effect on the muscles and helps regulate heart rhythms. It even has a calming effect on the brain and can be especially helpful in decreasing heightened stress states often associated with anxiety.

I have learned that many Christians, particularly in Western culture, are a bit uncomfortable (if not terrified) by the subject of deep breathing exercises, and especially meditation. For them, meditation raises the concern that a demonic force or spirit will take residency in a mind that is emptied. Similar fears exist with the mention of the word "hypnosis."

Yet, with regards to meditation, by visualizing good things, the brain is re-programmed in like manner.

While there are a variety of styles of meditation, I personally prefer meditation exercises that are fixed on a particular quality or attribute, such as love.

This style of meditation is termed *kataphatic* meditation (a Greek term meaning, among other things, "intimate communication from the top down"). This is representative of biblical forms of meditation, such as what David practiced in meditating on God's character, creation, and provision when he wrote his psalms.

The ability to meditate effectively takes effort and discipline. The "muscles" of meditation must be strengthened. This can only be accomplished through practice.

Additionally, the benefits of meditation are in direct proportion to the amount of *time* (duration) that one is able to sustain attention, his or her *intensity* of focus, and the essential quality of the *object* upon which they meditate.

In terms of hypnosis, most people's fears are laid to rest when I explain that hypnosis is similar to when an athlete, upon focusing intently, might describe him or herself as being "in the zone" of peak performance. I then concede that just like any form of therapy, client safety is always proportionate to both the competence and professional ethics of the therapist.

I once had a client, Cathy, who suffered a rather severe form of automatic negative thoughts. Being that Cathy is a devout Christian, and due to matters of faith, during our initial sessions whenever I mentioned the terms "meditation" or "hypnosis" I observed her body position visibly shift, and her foot and leg begin to rock nervously, indicating uneasiness with these subjects. Upon noticing this, I discussed with Cathy the various forms of meditation and hypnosis, assuring her that the methods I use are not in any way in conflict with her faith, but rather, a potential enhancement to her faith and communication with God. She began to relax, and with her permission, we proceeded.

Recognizing that she is a devout student of the bible, and knowing something of that subject matter myself, I led her through a series of relaxation exercises with scriptural themes, e.g., meditating on the promises of God for her life.

We agreed that whenever an intrusive thought would come to mind, she would write it in her journal (she kept it with her at all times), and then immediately counteract it with a scriptural promise, i.e., a more truthful representation of God's will and intentions for her life. At the end of the day, she would compile the ANT themes (there are typically a few root themes within which negative thoughts cluster) and write each one on a clean sheet of paper. Then she would leave a few empty lines below the negative thought-cluster wherein she could write positive counteracts based on promises of scripture. By the end of the day, she had positive, more truthful messages to implant into her mind. She would rehearse and meditate on these before going to bed, and then again the following morning before heading out for the day.

The exercise looks something like this:

CLEAN SHEET OF PAPER

NAME   DATE

Negative thought cluster one - I will never be well.

Counteracted by - Someday I will be whole. I may not know when that will be, but I will follow my doctor's suggestions, make reasonable health choices and seek for a cure. In the meantime, I will trust God when He says, "Behold, I make all things new. . . . There will be no more illness," someday.

She then practiced visualizing herself healed, enjoying the freedom of mobility and skipping about freely and joyously. She allowed her mind to experience what that will be like. She invited all of her five senses to the party and had fun with it. She also rehearsed the many things she was able do in her present situation, and was prompted to identify the ways in which this time in her life could be reframed for good.

Negative thought cluster two - I will always be alone. I am unable to make friends because I was never taught how to be appropriately assertive.

Counteracted by - I am a gentle, loving, and intelligent woman. I have a lot to offer in friendship and to a community. I will enhance my social skills and learn to be more assertive.

She then meditated on a related scripture passage and visualized herself with friends and as an active member of her faith and neighborhood communities.

Each of these positive counteracts was then reinforced by daily practical steps towards achieving her goals.

It is amazing how these exercise enhanced Cathy's walk with God. She no longer felt shackled, bitter toward God, and thus, *dry* in her faith. Instead, her faith really came *alive* as she put God's promises into practice.

These exercises are powerful faith builders, and great for programming positive thought scaffolds.

Healing Painful Memories

Processing and Reorganizing Memories

This is a specific exercise that is best done with a trained psychotherapist or hypnotherapist, because it requires skilled guidance for maximum benefit and safety. Also, the nurturing quality of the therapist often plays a crucial role in the healing process.

This exercise is best described in the story of Anil (Session Four).

Additional Considerations

Diet - It is now common knowledge that "you are what you eat." This is especially true with reference to the health of your brain. The brain's nerves and fibers are healthy in direct proportion to the food that you consume. Too much sugar, tobacco products, alcohol, stress, and a host of other toxin producing substances, impact the physical structure of the brain, and hence, its performance. For more on this, I defer to neuroscientists and medical doctors specializing in this area.

Medication - People often ask about medication and its impact on the body and brain. Again, I defer to a medical doctor on this subject. However, research seems to indicate a positive correlation between medication and treatment effectiveness in many instances. It is wise to consult your physician with regards to weighing the potential side effects and benefits of medication.

Some physicians prefer a conservative approach to medication. While recognizing the benefits of medication, they might also recommend natural supplements to assist in healing the brain in certain cases.

Counseling and Therapy - As this book has stated clearly from the beginning, the ideas, suggestions, and techniques offered herein are not a replacement for psychotherapy.

While it is true that many of these exercises can be completed by you with potentially great benefits, individuals who suffer symptoms of a clinical nature should seek professional help right away.

Community - In our fast-paced culture, community is an all-too-often forgotten concept. Powerful things happen in community. Whether it is a small group, a church, a community support program, or a coaching and mentoring situation, community can provide powerful healing and opportunities for personal growth. Many of the world's most successful people attribute their success to the power of community, as well as personal or small group mentoring.

Interestingly enough, group therapy is often credited as being among the most effective forms of therapy in terms of client progress and reported relief of symptoms.

In light of research regarding the need for increased therapist-to-community involvement, more and more therapists are responding by increasing their involvement in the community, as well as conducting group therapy sessions.

Groups bring together the energy, wisdom, and support of people who are gathered for a common cause. For this reason, intensive group coaching is a service that I have increasingly incorporated into my practice.

There is strength in numbers!

SESSION SIX

GRADUATING COGNITIVE BOOT CAMP

Congratulations! With your cognitive mind care strategies fully in place, you are now ready to embark on the next leg of this exciting journey—a journey filled with exciting possibility, adventure, and discovery. This is where the cognitive portion of the New Mind Synergy (NMS = CG2) formula naturally transitions into the goals portion (Part Two). So get ready!

Thus far, you have learned many things about the mind related to the importance of maintaining it. As we begin the next part of the book, you will discover how clear cognition empowers you to more readily envision, step into, and realize your personal goals. Conversely, you will notice how goals serve to increase cognitive clarity. Each amplifies the other. This is New Mind Synergy at its best!

We have already reviewed what neuroscientists are saying about neuroplasticity and the ability for our brains to change and adapt. New Mind Synergy is further supported by scientific discoveries related to the systemic nature of various aspects of our universe (from micro- to macro- systems), insofar as a change in one component of a system often results in changes to other components as well. This information proves especially useful in highlighting the dynamic power of the New Mind Synergy formula as we shift into the following sessions.

As you read Part Two, related to goals, you may easily find yourself referring back to Part One. That is a good thing. It means you are taking it all in and understanding the relationship between your *cognitive thoughts* (Part One, primarily dealing with the conscious mind) and your *heart*, i.e., *mind, soul, and spirit* (Part Two, dealing a bit more with subconscious processes, e.g., attraction, goal setting, and visualization, etc.—but also with conscious processes too, e.g., planning, filtering, and analyzing information, etc.).

It is my hope that as you read, you will work through the exercises diligently. If you are at all like me, you may have a tendency to skip over them, preferring instead to simply read the book's contents.

A Word of Caution: The power of Get Up! New Mind Synergy lies in the practical application of the knowledge presented—working in tandem with the exercises. Please do not skip the exercises, as they will assist you in applying what you are learning. To the degree that you apply this formula, you will grow and progress.

Also, consider asking yourself the following questions:

One - What have I learned thus far about my thoughts and how my brain works?

Two - What are some areas of my life wherein I have been held back from growing because of my, what Zig Ziglar and many in the recovery movement refer to as, "stinkin' thinkin'"?

Three - Which exercises from Part One (cognition) did I especially find helpful? How can I apply what I have learned to my life, beginning right now?

I am rooting for you as you embark on this next step towards wholeness and life success!

Part Two

Goals!

(Putting the "G" in New Mind Synergy = CG^2)

"give me a 'g'!"

$$\text{NMS} = \text{CG}^2$$

New Mind Synergy

Session Seven

Goals!

Success is goals. The rest is commentary.

-Brian Tracy

In this session, your new *cognitive* mind set (conscious mind, *thoughts*, Part One) and the power of *goals* (subconscious mind, *intuition, emotion, inspiration* and *imagination*, Part Two) will converge, resulting in the dynamic integration of two distinct, yet interrelated, elements of *you*. You will discover that clean *cognition* clears the runway of your mind, while *goals* tap into motivation, by fueling your personal power, resulting in the dynamic, life-changing force that is New Mind Synergy.

Your Moment to Break Free

While I do not know the particulars of your situation and what it is that you may be currently facing, e.g., a failed business or marriage, an estranged child, the ravages of a natural disaster, economic misfortune, self-destructive patterns of behavior, bondage to an addiction, loneliness, or any other number of potential difficulties—there is one thing that I do know for sure—the past is gone and it is now time to break free and begin rebuilding your life!

The past is a memory, the future a dream, today is a gift—that is why it is called the present.

-Unknown

Do Not Ever Give Up!

Successful people view personal mistakes, failures, and misfortune as opportunities to learn, grow, and improve their methods en route to success. They do not give up. Even though they may have failed at something, they themselves are not failures, because they are still trying hard in the push towards their goals. Hopefully, you will adopt a similar mindset.

Drawing a Line in the Sand

History tells us that in 168 B.C., a Roman Consul named Gaius Popillius Laenas drew a circular line in the sand around King Antiochus IV of the Seleucid Empire, then commanded, "Before you cross this circle, I want you to give me a reply for the Roman Senate"—the implication was that Rome would declare war should the King step out of the circle before making a commitment to leave Egypt immediately. After considering his options, the King decided to withdraw (this was probably a very wise move, as historians tell us that defeat was all but certain) and the Romans effectively accomplished their objective without the spilling of blood.

One important key to success lies in developing the ability to draw lines in the sand consistent with your values for living. This means strengthening your willingness to let go of the people, places, and things that will potentially bring you down. These kinds of decisions and commitments require courage and decisiveness.

Perhaps you can recall the saying, "no guts—no glory!" This adage holds true especially in relationship to life decisions, and the lines that must be drawn to strengthen them. Lines of decision can range from seemingly little sacrifices, such as, leaving the party at a decent hour in order to ensure proper rest for the next day's responsibilities, to leaving behind a relationship that is unhealthy and damaging to your personal growth and success—though you may have to endure some tears and moments of loneliness as a down payment towards a better, future reward.

"What Do I *Truly* Want?"

This once again begs the central question, "What do I *truly* want for my life?" If you could take a magic pill (see Session Five) and suddenly create any life that you want, what would your life look like? Would one of your desires be to live free of the cognitive roots of failure that have sabotaged your success for all of these years? What problems would be resolved? What would you set out to accomplish that has always seemed impossible for you? What kind of person would you like to become?

Uprooting the Old, Beginning Anew

As we progress throughout the remainder of the book, some of the common roots of failure (Session Two) will likely surface in your mind. You might ask, "Why would these emerge just as I am beginning to focus on my life goals?" The answer lies in the fact that they represent your former manner of living, i.e., a very real part of the way you *use* to think about, see, and do things. But don't worry. As you refer back to Session Five (Growing a Healthy Mind Forrest) and apply the techniques so useful in destroying these cognitive stumbling blocks, while simultaneously forging ahead towards establishing a goals blueprint for life success, you will discover that the soil is beginning to loosen beneath your feet, and that what once held you back is beginning to be uprooted—this is New Mind Synergy, a cognition and goals combination, beginning to perform its work in your life!

So, let's dig in . . .

The Power of Goals

So sure of the power of goals, that after years of speaking with audiences all over the world about personal transformation and success, world renowned motivational speaker, author, and entrepreneur, Brian Tracy, says, "If I was only given five minutes to speak to you, and I could only convey one thought that would help you to be more successful, I would tell you to write down your goals, make plans to achieve them, and work on your plans every single day." He continues, "This advice, if you followed it, would be of more help to you than anything you could ever learn" (Tracy, 2003).

In expressing this sentiment, Brian Tracy is certainly not alone. In fact, many of the most successful people in the world, representing a broad range of endeavors, equate the power of goals as a key component to their success. A small sample of such people includes the following: Abigail Adams, Dale Carnegie, Dorothea Dix, Thomas Edison, Ella Fitzgerald, Henry Ford, Harvey Firestone, Charles M. Schwab, late President Woodrow Wilson, and F.W. Woolworth.

Psychology research reveals that goals infuse an individual with a sense of meaning, purpose, and motivation—all important elements of personal happiness and success.

The greatest need of the human being is to have a sense of meaning and purpose in life.
-Viktor Frankl

The Many Positive Benefits of Goals

There are many positive benefits to a goals-centered life, expressed as follows:

Anticipation and curiosity - a byproduct of goals resulting in a positive and heightened state of vigilance. This state causes increased activity in the attentional areas of the brain, including the reticular cortex. Anticipation and curiosity are known as "appetitive states" because they stimulate the mind's appetite, and hence, are highly motivating.

Research shows that anticipation of receiving or achieving something positive increases the consistent transmission of neuro-chemical resources necessary to maintain focused attention. It is under such conditions that we are apt to thrive and be at our best. In fact, the anticipation of positive events ". . . drives up the pleasure in the brain even more than the reward itself" (Shultz, Dayan, & Montague, 2002).

Positive energy, personal empowerment (dynamite or *dunamis* as a Greek equivalent), *increased confidence, competence,* and *inspired motivation* are all additional byproducts of the goals-centered life. In fact, I often describe goals as "fuel in the engine of life," sparking increased enthusiasm, personal satisfaction, and just plain old fun!

Additionally, goals are personally very *anchoring*, as they provide a positive and focused structure for your mind and for the direction of your life. It would be quite difficult to make a careless, foolish, potentially life- altering decision after having first consulted your very own personal goals blueprint for life success!

Finally, goals *simplify*. By establishing clearly defined goals for your life ahead of time, you will not have to spend precious time and energy agonizing about every decision that comes your way. You will already have the answers. When an opportunity presents itself, you simply compare it with your goals. If the opportunity is consistent with your goals and vision for life, then your decision is essentially already made. If not, then you can reject it without ever looking back, resulting in a definitive crispness to the way you manage your life.

Why Do So Few Harness the Power of Goals?

The concept of goals is nothing new. In fact, it has been written and spoken about perhaps more than any other topic of which I am aware— particularly within motivational literature. And yet, surprisingly, a relatively small number of people actually incorporate goals into their lives in any sort of consistent manner.

Most people have a desire to be happy, but no real plan on how to get what it is they say they want. Therefore, desire remains nothing more than a wish, hope, or dream. Wishing and hoping that things will get better is simply not enough!

Mark H. McCormack, in his book *What They Don't Teach You at Harvard Business School* tells of a Harvard study conducted between 1979 and 1989. At the beginning of the study, graduates of the Harvard MBA program were asked if they had clear, written goals for their future, and plans on how their goals would be accomplished. As it turns out, only three percent of the graduates had written goals, while thirteen percent had goals, but not written. The remaining sample of students had no concrete goals beyond the activities of daily life. Ten years later, the members of that same class were interviewed again, and it was revealed that those who had goals (but not written) earned twice as much money as those with no goals. And the three percent who had clear and written goals were earning (on average) ten times the amount of money as the other ninety-seven percent of graduates!

With such a marked difference between the relatively few who set goals, and those who do not, why do so few people set clear, specific, time-bound goals?

This remains somewhat of a mystery, but here are some possible reasons:

1. *Most people are not trained to set goals* – and for reasons unbeknownst to me, goals are not often emphasized in our current culture in any real focused way. This sparks the following question: could it be that our culture has become so comfortable and numb to the struggles of life (I am reminded of what our forefathers endured at the founding of this great nation, and then again through the great depression of the 1930s), that we take far too much for granted?

Could political correctness and the hesitancy to introduce anything to students that might be construed (even if remotely) as values-laden (within the overall framework of our educational system) be the reason that goals are not emphasized? And would the subject of goals be considered values-laden or values-neutral anyway?

In final analysis, since it currently stands that high school and college students are likely to complete their programs in the typical American college and university of today without any real formal exposure to the benefits of living a goal-centered life, it appears that parents, together with the movers-and-shakers of today, will have to be the educators in this regard.

But that's okay! Because the movers-and-shakers of today are easy to identify, as follows: they sell records, make media appearances, influence our culture by helping to shape public opinion and policy, discover scientific breakthroughs, serve those in need with bravery and courage, and create jobs—the entrepreneurs—those living the lives that so many of us enjoy watching on reality television!

You might ask, "Can a goals-centered life really make a significant difference for me personally? Can I really make a significant impact on my culture?" The answer resides, at least in part, in Orison Swett Marden's ground-breaking work, *Pushing to the Front* (1894), as well as another motivational classic, Napoleon Hill's *Think and Grow Rich* (1937).

These works (and a handful of other inspirational writings) are credited with inspiring a nation of men and women to greatness through such perilous times as the Great Depression and two world wars. Together with other important socio-cultural and political variables in play during this difficult time, motivational literature helped form the catalyst for what would later become a triumphant American comeback. Indeed, much of the prosperity that we now enjoy as a nation resulted from these pivotal early twentieth-century decades in American history.

Our Nation Stands at a Crossroads

Today our nation stands at a crossroads once again. With debilitating economic conditions staring us in the face, and a long-term financial forecast that is increasingly grim, the future of America (as we know it) weighs in the balance.

Some religious scholars interpret a mysterious absence of the United States of America in the closing scenes of the book of Revelation as proof positive that the U.S. will ultimately become a neutralized entity on the world scene. Could this actually happen? If so, what would likely be the cause? Could an inability to get our financial "house in order" contribute to the destruction of the greatest nation the world has ever known? Let's hope not. However, I personally believe that our current financial threats are very real.

That is precisely why we need our modern day heroes to emerge—heroes just like *you*—creative visionaries who possess the courage and conviction to aim high, placing principle above greed by obtaining wealth honestly, and never on the backs of others.

Now is a Great Time to Get Started

Now, perhaps more than ever, is a great time to make your mark on the world: whether it is getting your message out (via the internet, social media, radio, television, newspaper, or personal networking); lending your services to those in need; or starting your own business and creating jobs that will help stimulate the economy, there arguably has never been a more important time than now.

Great Leaders are Forging the Way

Recent advances in human studies have sparked the dawn of a new era. What is often termed the "self-help" or "Human Motivation Movement" is witnessing the rise of young superstars who have become entrepreneurs, educators, authors, life coaches, business marketing and innovations experts—people who make it their profession to assist others towards discovering what was helpful for them—namely, the power of desire, creativity, intuition, perseverance, and the goals-centered life.

The likes of leading marketing expert, entrepreneur, business and life success coach Alexandria Brown of Ali International; Tory Johnson, Good Morning America career expert and founder of *Women for Hire* (attracting talented women and leading employers); business consultant and social influencer Kristin Andress; entrepreneur and success coach James Malinchak; business and organizational development expert Dr. Susan Murphy; internet marketing guru, Terri Romine, of 1 Net Marketing Service; and life coach, community leader, and mover-and-shaker, Coaching to Vision's Jasenka Sabanovic; together with many others. These all serve as shining examples of leaders who, having starting from scratch, are inspiring others with their courage and passion for helping a generation achieve great things. What role will you play?

Coaching in Culture

As a culture, we need to begin thinking less of tolerating mediocrity and merely containing problematic (or low) cognitive function, and more in terms of stimulating greatness (of purpose, action, and thought) if we intend on rising once again to the crescendo of greatness that mark's our nation's heritage. We must become specialists in the potentiality of human endeavor.

Imagine if a significant percentage of Americans alive today would practice the principles of this book wholeheartedly. What sort of changes do you imagine might take place within our culture? Indeed, the implications for your personal life (specifically) and for our culture (more broadly) are astounding.

A Unique Moment in Time

This is a unique moment in the coaching profession, as life coaches are poised to offer tremendous benefit to those clients who truly desire life transformation. Your personal survival, as well as our national survival, just may depend on it!

Digging Deeper

Financial security stripped for a season, many are discovering the need to dig deeper than ever before, to move out of their comfort zone, and embrace the very best of what they have to offer to those within their sphere of influence.

In times past (the days of our founding as a nation), greatness was spawned from a desperate need to survive, as well as a desire for a better life. It is only within the past several decades that this desperation-spawned creative passion has been lost. We have become a comfortable and often valueless culture (lack of morals corrupts effective industry). We need to rediscover our heritage and pension for soulful living, hard work, and industry.

Now is the Time. America, Get Up!

Now is a particularly good time for this to occur, because sometimes the greatest of opportunities abound in a struggling economy. We need to capitalize on the abundance of opportunities before us. The time for building is now, so let's Get Up! and get moving.

2. *Fear of failure* - as discussed in The Cognitive Roots of Failure, Session Two.

3. *Desire for security* - we must remember that success (and its accompanying security) is achieved by those individuals who are willing to step out of their comfort zone and take risks (as discussed in the Cognitive Roots of Failure, Session Two).

Those who courageously take steps to fulfill their destiny are the ones likely to fare best in the decades to come, especially as our nation's middle class socioeconomic standing (due to increasing national debt, higher taxes, inflation, and job and economic uncertainty) provides an increasingly less desirable lifestyle option (more on this in Session Ten).

4. *Contentment with the status quo* - is merely a polite way of suggesting that people often settle for less than their best.

Our Hidden Genius

Each of us has a special gift—a hidden genius. We must amplify this gift through goals if we are to ever reach the levels of success that are possible.

Many people possess a hidden genius that remains untapped. As I wrote earlier—frustration, confusion, and depression result to the extent this is the case.

If you happen to be waiting for something or someone in order to begin establishing goals for your life, then really only this question remains: For what and for whom are you waiting?"

Truthfully, the only one who can make *your* life happen the way *you* want it is *you*!

How Goals Changed My Life

After serving as a counselor and seminar presenter for nine years, in 2004 I experienced what is often termed, "career burnout." On reflecting, I have identified three contributing factors to my struggle at that time: (*i*) personal and professional immaturity, (*ii*) limited personal financial compensation, and finally, (*iii*) lack of clearly defined career goals. Surprisingly, my burnout had very little, if anything, to do with the typical hazards of listening to people's problems (as is ordinarily the case for mental health workers in relation to professional burnout).

Sadly enough, I did not have clearly defined goals *because I was never trained in this way*. Therefore, although I was able to help quite a few people, had established a successful seminar and workshop series, and even managed to complete a portion of my doctoral studies (all by the age of twenty-eight), I was not yet equipped with the personal and professional tools necessary to take my career to the next level. My skill-set (and my income with it) had hit an anti-climatic plateau.

Therefore, since according to my high school senior year aptitude tests (remember those?), my second highest score was in sales and customer service (the first was counseling—surprise! surprise!), I decided to go into commission-based retail sales, just to shake things up a bit while I figured out my future plans. I remained in retail sales for nearly four years, just enough time to learn some skills that would prove invaluable for my future.

Interestingly enough, my venture into sales is where I was first introduced to the power of *goals*, as well as many other important lessons that would prove crucial for life success in the years to come.

I first learned about goals through a sales trainer by the name of Mark Thomas. We all called him "Coach." Coach had played basketball in college and was brought up through the ranks by the coach-of-all-coaches, the late Coach John Wooden of UCLA. Since Coach Wooden was known for his "basics and fundamentals" style of coaching, Mark taught his new sales staff in very much the same manner. Since Mark had managed to make a high six-figure income for many years as a sales professional, I figured he knew what he was talking about. So I listened, learned, and applied all that I could.

During that time, I learned that success is determined not so much by personal talent (although talent is a factor to some degree), but rather, by setting and consistently pursuing clearly defined personal sales goals.

Those who followed a plan and worked it consistently were ultimately the most successful in sales.

For instance, take those earning two hundred thousand, three hundred thousand, or even five hundred thousand dollars per year in retail sales commissions—these represent two to three percent of sales professionals—I found that they are not superstars any more than you or I (or the neighbor, Joe, living down the street for that matter). They simply followed super-star methods of applying relatively simple, but crucial procedures in their sales game plan. Hmmm, much like life!

They envision what they want, set goals, intensely and consistently focus on their goals, become knowledgeable about their product, and serve their clients well—they under-promise and over-deliver—maintaining a long term business outlook.

Maintaining a long-term business outlook, they are not merely interested in the "home run" deal, but rather, in earning customer loyalty over the long-haul.

Therefore, they are honest, hardworking, and willing to do the seemingly little things that others are not, e.g., sending birthday and holiday cards to their customers, or sending a special gift in recognition of an important moment in their customer's life. In essence, they convey a genuine personal interest in their customers.

As I studied the characteristics of some of the top retail sales producers in the nation, I quickly learned that natural talent is further down the list of success attributes than many people realize. In fact, honesty, product knowledge, attention to customer needs and wants, a personal touch, and a set of clearly defined professional goals remain at the very top of the list.

Having applied all that Coach taught me, I managed to more than double my income in those four years, broke numerous sales records, and quickly rose to a sales manager position. I even managed to work for a national corporation wherein I was afforded a luxury personal automobile, extravagant client entertainment expense account, and travels to various cities (always via limousine from the airport), as well as accommodations at some of the nation's finest hotels.

Truthfully, I felt as if I had gone "from rags to riches" in a relatively short period of time, and all because of the power of goals, combined with consistently working a very basic system that reflected those goals.

However, my heart was calling me back to my first love, that of counseling, speaking, and writing. Fortuitously, I was able to hand off my sizeable customer following to someone I felt would take good care of "my people."

With some of my knowledge gaps about business (and the way the world works) filled in, and armed with a clear understanding of the power of goals, I was ready to embrace my career once again, but this time in a more intentional, and therefore, effective way.

Take Courage!

I share this tidbit about my life realizing that many people's lives have been overturned by the economic struggles currently facing our nation. I wish to convey hope.

I started with virtually nothing, and was able to make significant strides quickly—all of which I attribute to the power of goals, together with a positive attitude, and intense desire.

Show me a really great triumph that is not the reward of persistence. Genius, when you look more closely at it, usually turns out to be the sum of uncommon dedication to a task.

-Orison Swett Marden

Winding Roads Sometimes Lead You Home

Also, I share this personal information to illustrate how virtually everything in our lives (even winding roads!) can contribute towards building the foundation of our success—if we will but listen, learn, and apply the lessons as we go.

Go. Move. Just Get Started!

We do not have to wait to have it all figured out before getting started. The truth is, we will *never* have it all figured out. That is why Woody Allen is quoted as having said, "80 percent of success is just showing up." The hardest part is getting started.

What about You?

What has your life been like to this point? What experiences (*victories* and *failures*) have you encountered that might serve as a foundation of wisdom towards strengthening your ability to move forward with increased power and confidence? You will want to list these as a reference for Session Ten.

What about Right Now?

Are you presently going through the throes of a life-altering circumstance or tragic situation? If so, are you struggling to see beyond the clouds of confusion, bitterness, and despair—in hopes of discovering a brighter tomorrow? How can this experience—the tilling of your heart's soil, the lessons learned, and the skills developed—serve as a foundation for future success? You will want to list these as well.

As posed by the question in the book's Introduction, *Could this dark night of the soul serve as a curious beckoning, calling you to explore untapped reservoirs of possibility that have lay dormant within you all along? Could this book offer clues that will assist you in discovering many of the answers to your life's disappointments, launching you on a journey of personal success and fulfillment beyond anything you could have ever imagined?*

I invite you to consider that it is not so much what happens to us, but what we glean from it, that ultimately determines success.

In the Sessions Ahead—Application!

In the sessions ahead, you will learn many of the best strategies for success—strategies I have studied ever since that transformational period in my life (2004-2007)—you will envision a better life, attract more of what it is that you truly want, set goals centered around your personal vision, and then implement the kinds of qualities and characteristics that will help to ensure your success.

Good luck getting started!

SESSION EIGHT

VISION

Where there is no vision, the people perish.
-Proverbs 29:18

Vision allows us to see with our mind's eye what it is that we truly want, before it becomes a reality. Some would even argue that once something is envisioned—*it is reality*—we just need to begin walking in, talking in, and making decisions in accordance with this new reality.

It is fascinating to think that at the moment we envision something, with a sincerity, passion, desire, and determination so strong that we will do whatever is necessary to see it manifest in the physical world, that at that very moment, marching orders have been sent throughout the cosmos. Then, it is only a matter of time before we see with our own eyes that which our mind has already seen.

Such was the case with Walt Disney when many decades ago he envisioned a family theme park that would be "The Happiest Place on Earth." There is a sign at the Epcot Center in Orlando Florida that quotes Disney, "If you can dream it, you can do it."

Of course at the time that he first envisioned his theme parks, it was just that, a vision. Or was it?

Present Realization

One of the strongest tools of which I am personally aware is what I call *present realization*. Present realization is when you hold a vision in your mind's eye of something that you want to manifest in your life. It may be a material object, such as, a new sports car; a certain lifestyle; an award or level of academic or professional achievement; a trophy for winning a prestigious event; a character quality or personality characteristic; or any number of things that you desire.

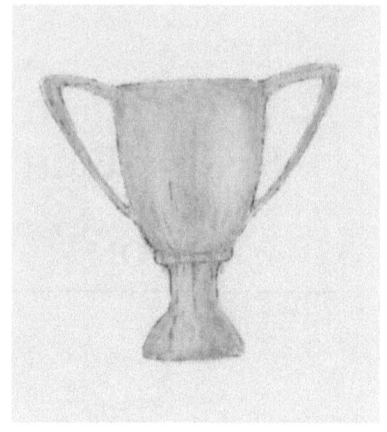

For present realization to be effective, it must emanate from within. It must be something that you desire in your heart of hearts. Also, it must be intense enough to captivate your senses and occupy your thoughts. You will see it, smell it, touch it, taste it, and hear it. For example, a golfer aspiring to win the championship in a prestigious tournament might visualize himself calm, relaxed, and swinging at his very best—"in the zone" of peak performance. He will feel the metal of the trophy as he raises it high into the air, hear the crowd chanting his name, see fans' faces full of glee, taste the champagne and chocolate-covered strawberries at the club house reception, and smell the leather of the new car he just won as he pulls out of the club house and heads back home—a winner!

Present realization lies in the *duration, frequency, intensity,* and *vividness* of your vision (Tracy, 2003). It is good to practice present realization on a daily basis—focusing on one, two, or three primary goals at a time. I often use it to ensure a successful day and for power to knock through challenges that seem to be in my way at any given moment in time. Also, I use it for long- term goals as a tool to guide my mind towards the realization of where it is I want to go in the future.

Present realization is an exercise with tremendous potential for personal transformation, as it allows you to experience—see, smell, touch, taste, and hear—the very attainment (and it's sweet fruit!) toward which you are aspiring.

Present realization is personally invigorating. It attunes your mind to a heightened level of success and personal experience, and thus, becomes a very real part of your minds DNA—to the point where you would never want to settle for less than your personal best.

Another great benefit of Present Realization is that by infusing your life with the very thoughts and feelings that accompany the success-laden and enjoyable events being envisioned, you increasingly integrate a success mind-set and begin to realize that it is just a matter of time before what you are seeking manifests in physical form.

It is often said that happiness is not a destination, but very much a real part of the journey. With this in mind, why not begin enjoying (walking in) your success right now?

It All Started with a Vision

Dr. Susan Murphy, business and organizational development expert, shares a remarkable story about her father who, many years ago, borrowed money from his father-in-law and moved 700 miles from Maryland to Atlanta, Georgia, with a vision for starting a heating and air conditioning company from scratch. She recalls, "He never wavered from his vision. In fact, when he found a shortage of engineers in Atlanta, he set up a university program to train students. . . . Despite enormous set-backs, when the company burned down, and when two of the key salesman were critically injured in a traffic accident, he kept the vision. Years later he sold the company, but at customer request, kept working until well into his 80's" (Insight Pub., 2004).

Dr. Murphy then goes on to share about the teachings of Dr. Peter Senge, as a complement to the research of Dr. Bennis, wherein he taught her "the importance of having a clear vision of where you want to go," and "about the 'structural tension' that occurs when you think about your vision (or where you want to be) and your current reality. The farther your vision is from your current reality, the higher the tension level—and the greater the discomfort. To decrease this 'structural tension' you can either move your current reality (your current state) toward your vision or lower your vision (your goals) to be closer to your current reality. We often will lower our goals because that's easier" (Insight Pub., 2004).

She then draws an illustration from her life's work wherein she and Dr. Pat Heim were in the midst of "mounds of research" for a new book addressing the "challenges and opportunities women face when working with other women," and found the volume of research involved to be a bit taxing, "stressful and uncomfortable." Nevertheless, enduring through the process, they achieved their publishing goals, and their book, *In the Company of Women* (2001) has been so successful, that it has been published in several different languages. It all started with a vision! (Insight Pub., 2004).

The ancestor of every action is thought.

-Ralph Waldo Emerson

What is your vision?

In Session Ten, you will have a chance to transplant your personal vision into your goals blueprint. So why not "swing for the fence?" After all, you only live once!

Action Steps

Write answers to the following questions using the space provided below.

Q 1. What are some things you are currently aspiring to? And how can entering into *present realization* help you achieve or realize these goals in your life today?

Q 2. What differences can *present realization* make in your behavior and attitude right now?

Q 3. How can *present realization* and the power of visualization make a difference in the one thing that you presently struggle with the most?

Complete this *present realization* exercise:

Envision one thing that you really want to see manifest in your life. Allow sufficient time for your mind to see, hear, smell, touch, and/or taste the accomplishing of that goal.

Write your feelings and observations in the space provided below:

SESSION NINE

LAW OF ATTRACTION

All that we are is the result of what we have thought.

-Buddha

To understand the law of attraction, it is important to first understand our surroundings.

This was first made plain to me while studying systems theory at both the micro- and macro- levels, and learning that everything in the universe consists of the same thing—energy. Everything we consider as solid matter—from the automobile we drive to the chair we rely on to withstand our weight—consists merely of a bunching of molecules of atoms separated by gaps of space. Looking through a high-powered microscope, we would see atoms consisting of a nucleus with protons spinning around them—much like planets spinning around the sun.

But since we naturally experience our bodies in this physical realm in somewhat limited dimensions, we must stretch ourselves to remain mindful that our perception is equally limited, and that a realm quite independent of physical matter, and in many ways quite superior to physical matter, exists. The fact is, we are energy, including our thoughts. With this in mind, the law of attraction becomes increasingly tenable.

Since as humans we consist of energy (much like the proton spinning around the nucleus) our thoughts can be either positive or negative. And since our thoughts are powerful, they effectively transmit either positive or negative energy into the universe, and receive like kind in similar proportion via the law of attraction. Hence the common saying, "That which you sow, shall you also reap."

Energy and Relationships

Centuries-old traditions examining attraction and compatibility suggest a correlation between similar energy (with reference to positive versus negative, and frequencies of energy) and degrees of relational happiness and success. It is often said that "opposites attract." While this may be true to some degree on a soul level—hence the term "soul-mate"—energy attraction, in terms of similar qualities, i.e., positive versus negative, and frequencies of energy, may potentially be regarded as a more substantial determining factor in achieving long-term relationship success.

Positive Versus Negative Attraction

If I am basically a positive person, then I will attract into my life positive circumstances and people. On the other hand, if I am basically a negative person, then I will attract into my life negative circumstances and people.

"For the thing which I greatly feared is come upon me . . . " (Job 3:25). This verse of scripture may provide a powerful example of how we attract that to which we pay much attention. Clearly, as this passage indicates, Job did not *want* calamity (the complete destruction of his entire household), but *focused* on it nonetheless. Therefore, his desire was out of harmony with his thoughts, which resulted in tragedy.

additionally (as the context of the story of Job makes clear) there were unseen spiritual forces working behind the scenes, engaged in a showdown of cosmic proportion.

Is The Law of Attraction for Real?

It would be unwise to dismiss the law of attraction as merely a hocus-pocus concoction of wishful dreamers distilling their own whimsical version of reality, as some may speculate. But rather, it appears to be a legitimate and powerful means through which countless men and women throughout the centuries, upon harnessing its raw power just prior to unleashing it as a driving force for good, have accomplished enormous feats. The book *Think and Grow Rich* (1937) recounts many such instances.

Some people ask, "What does the law of attraction mean, and what are the avenues of the mind through which this force works?"

Reticular Cortex

The reticular cortex is a finger-like section of the brain that deletes most of what you hear, see, and feel. It directs incoming stimulus to your conscious and subconscious mind. That is because at any given moment, there may be numerous things competing for your attention—both from within (your own head), and from without (your environment). However, if you were somehow forced to focus on them all at once, you could easily become overwhelmed.

The reticular cortex acts similar to a "gatekeeper" to help direct your attention, which enables you to focus on objects of primary importance to you at any given point in time. Therefore, the power of the reticular cortex lies mainly in its ability to direct, and therefore harness, your focus, attention, and intent.

Well directed effort is sometimes required to obtain an objective of desire. For example, if I intend to invest in a piece of property in town for a competitive price, I will have to conduct research regarding various locations, become familiar with local zoning laws, and contact a real estate professional for advice. This "due diligence" consists of things that I must do to secure the best possible outcome and achieve what it is that I desire. Otherwise, my intention is nothing but a mere wish or fantasy. As they say, "the road to hell is paved with good intentions." Therefore, it is the effort, preparation, and action surrounding intentionality that fosters a successful outcome—the accomplishment of one's goal.

Prepared people are lucky more often.

-Unknown

I have used the tool of intentionality numerous times, and with notable success. In fact, I can say that virtually every noteworthy endeavor that I have ever accomplished has involved the proper use of my reticular cortex, hard work, the cooperation of the universal law of attraction, and ultimately, the blessing of God.

A Practical Example

A couple of years ago, I heard about a local businessman who had an intense desire to reach out to the homeless people in his community. He did not have much to offer personally, but established a goal of feeding and clothing one hundred people per month from his little business property located in the center of town.

He obtained the proper permits, made up some flyers, ran an ad in the local newspaper asking for donations of everything from clothing and canned goods to kitchenware and volunteers, and met his goal of serving the homeless within several months. It is my belief that it all started with an intense desire to benefit others, and was accomplished via the proper use of his reticular cortex.

A man is what he thinks about all day long.
-Ralph Waldo Emerson

In his Ultimate Goals Program, entrepreneur, author, and internationally acclaimed motivational speaker, Brian Tracy, also speaks of a natural goal achieving mechanism, which enables a person to accomplish his or her desires according to the size, scope, and nature of the goals upon which he or she dwells (Tracy, 2003).

Tracy contends that by not only wanting something, but focusing on it (*duration, frequency, intensity,* and *vividness*) intensely, there seems to be a sense in which a person attracts the very thing that he or she is seeking. It is as if the universe begins to coordinate with his or her efforts and rallies around the attainment of the goal, ensuring that all necessary resources are brought together at the just the right time, and just the right place, for the realization of the desired objective (Tracy, 2003).

Man is a teleological organism.

-Aristotle

Tracy (2003), in teaching about the homing pigeon and its ability to find its way home, says,

You take a homing pigeon out of its roost, put it in a cage, cover the cage with a blanket, put the cage in a box, and then place the box into a closed truck cab. You can then drive a thousand miles in any direction. If you then open the truck cab, take out the box, take off the blanket, and let the homing pigeon out of the cage, the homing pigeon will fly up into the air, circle three times, and then fly unerringly back to its home roost a thousand miles away." He continues, *"This is the only creature on earth that has this incredible cybernetic, goal-seeking function in its brain, except for man. You have the same goal achieving ability as the homing pigeon, but with one marvelous addition. When you are absolutely clear about your goal, you don't even have to know where it is or how it is to be achieved. By simply deciding exactly what it is you want, you will begin to move unerringly towards your goal, and your goal will start to move unerringly towards you. At exactly the right time, and exactly the right place, you and the goal will meet.*

Man as a Teleological Being

While it is beyond the scope of this book to review the various philosophical, scientific, and theological implications of man's teleological connection to the universe, the truth remains that something powerful does indeed occur when intensity of focus is in alignment with the intent to achieve an objective. Beyond what I have already stated, in what manner it involves unseen, quantum physical occurrences, I am not personally sure. However, at minimum, it is clear that man is endowed by the Creator with the tools necessary to enhance his ability to focus the mind powerfully towards the accomplishment of significant feats.

Programming Success

Programming your mind for success (the success mind-set) with images and pictures of what you want is a very powerful practice. Once you have determined exactly what it is you want, then consider going to the store and buying magazines, newspaper articles, etc. and then clip and place the images and words that support your vision in places where you are likely to see them most often.

I wrote my vision on Post-Its and placed these Post-Its in strategic places, like my bathroom mirror, my desk drawer, and my Day-timer. I learned how important it is to write these characteristics in the present tense, as if I had already achieved them.

-Dr. Susan Murphy

Guard Your Associations

Finally, in relationship to the law of attraction, it is vitally important to be mindful of with whom and where you spend your time.

Negative people, places, and things will drain your vital energy and desire for success. Additionally, negative people will be prone to jealously criticize your progress.

On the other hand, positive people, places, and things will fuel your energy, and increase your desire for success.

Indeed, it is good to soar with other eagles. An eagle is someone soaring high, towards realizing great things in his or her life. Chances are an eagle will have strengths that you desire, and therefore, will encourage you towards greater heights of success than you might otherwise be able to obtain on your own.

To stimulate men and women to the discovery and perception of the truth— that they themselves are makers of themselves by virtue of the thoughts which they choose and encourage; that mind is the master-weaver, both of the inner garment of character and the outer garment of circumstance, and that, as they may have hitherto woven in ignorance and pain they may now weave in enlightenment and happiness.

-William James

Session Ten

Blueprint for Life Success

If you can imagine it, you can achieve it. If you can dream it, you can become it.

-William Arthur Ward

In a previous session, we reviewed the many positive benefits of goals. In this session, we will journey through a series of potentially life transforming exercises to help you get started with your new goals mind-set and blueprint for success.

A WORD OF CAUTION: *if you embrace and utilize the concepts and exercises laid-out in this session, you will likely never be the same. Your life will suddenly accelerate in a fast-forward motion. . . . So wear your seatbelt!*

Friends and family will stand amazed as they witness this awe-inspiring transformation taking shape.

The Need to Get Moving!

Forward acceleration of your life at this point in time just may not be such a bad idea. I write this for one simple reason—because the price is far too high to continue living in a haphazard manner!

Consider This

It used to be that if you were socioeconomically middle class, you could practically bump into a fifty to sixty thousand dollar per year salary (with paid benefits). If you managed your finances well, while this salary might not have afforded living in the lap of luxury, you could at least have lived a reasonably comfortable lifestyle, getting along pretty well. However, now with more people competing for fewer jobs, those days just may be gone, at least for the foreseeable future.

This dismal job outlook (combined with rising inflation, growing utility costs, skyrocketing gas prices, higher college and university tuition, and increased taxes) represents a real wake up call to the person planning on randomly conducting business as usual with regards to his or her economic future. Economists concerns about a shrinking middle class are consistent with economic data revealing an undeniably lower quality of life for the average American. Yes indeed, the days of "just winging it" seem to be over.

Who Will Thrive?

Individuals who are willing to create their own economic reality through innovation, courage, and creativity—fueled by clearly defined career and personal life goals—will march forth to claim the American dream in the twenty-first century.

Unfortunately, those who do not maintain this mind-set will likely see their quality of life (and that of their children and grandchildren) diminish markedly.

A Return to Our Roots is Needed, STAT!

To anyone who would reduce our culture and way of life via social policies of learned helplessness, the message is clear—Americans are a responsible, strong, "can-do" people! The spirit, courage, and ingenuity that made our nation great continue to reside within our blood!

However, we must be ever mindful that the window of opportunity may soon close if we do not all get moving, and quickly.

Calling All Heroes

In the U.S., there is a call for all heroes to emerge—people of firm conviction, enduring courage, and the vision necessary to reach great heights of success once again. Allow me to ask a couple of questions: Are you ready to access the hero in you? Are you ready to go for it and begin *really* living—life on the edge of your potential—perhaps even for the very first time?

We Must Avoid the Fate of Ancient Rome!

Otherwise we risk the fate of ancient Rome, who having been once great, was ultimately destroyed from within by similar threats to the decline of initiative and character that currently face our nation.

The minds of men were gradually reduced to the same level, the fire of genius was extinguished.
-History of the Decline and Fall of the Roman Empire

So, Get Up! and get moving. *Your family and country need you! You need you*!

Where to Begin

Fortunately, getting started and creating a goals blueprint for success is not anywhere close to rocket science. In fact, it is so simple that even a child can do it. Your goals should be so clearly stated that your neighbor's eight year old child can understand exactly what it is you want, and how you are going to get it. Remember, the power of goals does not rest on the complexity of the process, but rather, on the substantial passion you carry into any endeavor, the consistency with which you move forward, and the usability of the methods used for pursuing your goals.

Clarifying and Expanding Exercises

In the following, let's review the very best exercises to help you get started.

Magic Pill Technique - as discussed in Part One (please review in Session Five). This exercise represents a great place to start because it cuts right to the heart of what changes you would like to make in your life. It removes barriers to free thinking by suggesting that there is a "magic pill" that can remove anything that might try to stand in your way.

The Magic Pill Technique only requires that you have a sheet of paper, journal, or notebook. The "magic" in this exercise is of such a powerful variety that you could even scribble it onto a napkin while dining at a local café, and by merely reviewing it daily, still achieve amazing results. For these reasons, this is a great clarifying exercise.

I do suggest a notebook or some form of organizer for this and other exercises to follow, as you will want to build on these exercises in the days, weeks, months, and years to come.

One Page Miracle for the Soul - as discussed in Part One (please review in Session Five). This is another great exercise for helping to draw out your true values from deep within your soul.

Life's Last Days Question - involves asking yourself, "If I suddenly learned that I have a terminal illness, with only a matter of days, weeks, or months to live, what would I do with the remaining time?" This question will assist you towards quickly identifying your true values, i.e., what is really most important to you.

Also, you can ask, "What changes will I be making?" or "What relationships will I seek to mend?" or "With whom would I like to spend a majority of my time?" or "What kind of an impact would I like to make on those closest to me?" Perhaps there is a message that you would like to deliver to the world.

I especially like these questions, because they help put things into proper perspective. They are loaded with heart. For such reasons, they also represent great clarifying questions.

Why not consider living the rest of your life with this new mind-set?

Wish List - asks, "If you had no limitations at all, e.g., money, time, or health, what twenty-five to fifty goals would you most like to accomplish in your life?" I like this question because it helps us tap into some things we would enjoy doing, but have not paid much thought.

This is most definitely an expanding question, as it prompts an individual to think outside of the narrow confines of perceived limitations and routine thought, and invites exploration from a broadened perspective. With some creativity and careful consideration you will be amazed at how quickly you can come up with fifty, or even a hundred, things to include on your list.

What Do I Most Enjoy Doing? - asks the following question, "What would I do without pay if I could do only one thing all day long?" While this question can potentially lead an individual along the path of one-sided or imbalanced thinking, it would not likely be the case for very long, because he or she would soon realize that whatever they determine to do must also align with their core values with regards to the whole of life. So that, endless beer parties, poker, football games, and all night disco dancing would probably wear thin rather quickly. Besides, eventually someone will have to create a fresh round of alibis for the boss (and spouse!), pay the bar tab and DJ, and still have enough money left over to refresh the chips and salsa!

In all seriousness, this is another great clarifying question because it helps you identify that for which you are truly passionate and would most like to do with a good portion of your time.

Ask yourself, "What ways can I build more of what I truly love into my life?" For instance, if you dislike your present job, you might consider returning to school or volunteering some spare time to what you really love. You might also consider researching ways that you can effectively transition into your dream job.

Stirred or Shaken?

There is a joy that I have in sharing these techniques. It stems from the fact that I use them routinely and know firsthand what a powerful difference they can make in a person's life. In using them, do not be at all surprised if you begin to feel (as I did) a tremendous weight being lifted from your shoulders, and an emerging excitement full of wonder and possibility beginning to stir from deep within your heart and soul.

Follow the Steps Thoroughly . . . You Will Be Amazed!

When I created my own personal goals blueprint for life success, I followed the order of the five exercises as presented above. I pondered these clarifying and expansive questions thoroughly, realizing that they serve as an important prelude to effective life blueprint planning. Follow the steps thoroughly. You will be amazed. I am excited about your new journey of discovery.

The Basic Six

The Life Balance chart on the following page includes the six basic areas of life, and serves as a reminder to remain balanced and mindful of your core values while working through the exercises. *Note:* The One Page Miracle for the Soul exercise created by Dr. Daniel Amen (referred to in Session Five, and now here in Session Ten) identifies four broad categories of life to consider (with sub-categories beneath). The two charts are similar in content and principle one to another. I merely categorize mine a bit differently.

Life Balance

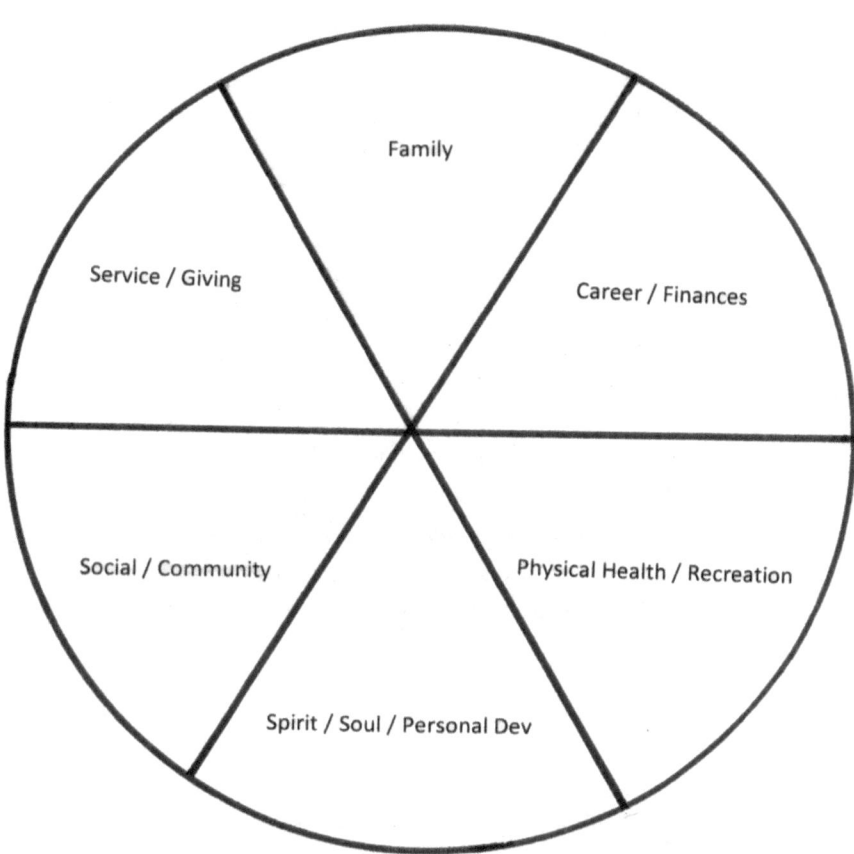

Life Success Blueprint

In this next section, I invite you to begin the next phase of synthesizing your goals into a clear and organized life success blueprint. It is best to organize your thoughts from general to specific, i.e., from *long-term goals (LTG)* to *short-term goals (STG)*—the opposite of how we typically organize our lives and daily activities. The reason is that you will want the long-term, "big picture," to inform the choices that you will be making in the near future. It would make little sense to chart short-term goals before first clarifying where it is that you ultimately wish to go.

Let's review each.

As noted in the Life Balance pie chart, long-term goals should reflect your values in terms of the following: social/community; spiritual/soul/ personal development; career/finances; family; physical health/recreation; and service/giving. These represent the six essential components of our lives.

*If you ignore even one major area of your life, it is then impossible to be truly whole. While balance may not be easy to achieve, it remains an important objective, as each component is interdependent one with another. For example, it would be unwise to tirelessly work eighty hours per week in pursuit of wealth, while leaving your family, personal health, and social life to suffer as a result.

After carefully considering the clarifying and expanding questions mentioned above, you will want to begin listing the long-term goals that emerge as a result of the process. I recommend combining various goals into one major goal whenever possible. For instance, if you have long-term goals of working for yourself, creating your own schedule, working from home, and managing your own professional development, then you would include these under a single, major long-term goal, entitled, "I Determine My Ideal Vocation and Working Conditions." (Remember, goals are best stated as personal, positive, and present tense—3P's.) The various sub-goals would then be listed beneath this one major goal, serving as a description of all this goal entails.

The next step is to identify the specific actions necessary to achieve this long-term goal. These actions become your short-term goals, and serve as stepping stones towards helping you achieve your ultimate objective(s).

Examples of short-term goals, together with what is often identified as your *Major Definite Purpose (MDP),* might be to obtain career counseling, conduct research to learn more about a career of interest, or saving the money required for training and/or business start-up costs. If you learned that you would need several thousand dollars for training and business start-up costs, but were currently unemployed and financially broke, then your major definite purpose (the one, two, or three things required to "get the ball rolling" and that would have the most immediate and substantial impact on your ability to move ahead towards your other goals) would be to obtain employment in something that does not require financial capital so that you can earn and save money as necessary to accomplish your short-term, and then eventually, your long-term goals.

In addition to being clear and specific, it is important that your goals be time-bound, so that your mind is alerted with an increased sense of urgency, for example: "I will obtain career counseling by such and such a date." When a date is set, your mind—via your reticular cortex—is alerted and begins to focus attention towards the goal, gathering the resources necessary for the attainment of the goal.

Remember, goals are meant to be accomplished. There is little value in setting goals that are unrealistic. Therefore, your goals must be achievable. Otherwise, you could become discouraged and quit. Reflecting on the illustrations about the king and builder (Part One, Session Two, "Clarity"), we realize that we must first determine what it is that we truly want, weigh the cost of obtaining it, and then decide whether or not to proceed.

Meet Patricia

As you read Patricia's story, see if you can identify the various stages of goal-setting and implementation.

The experience of a former client, Patricia, beautifully illustrates the progression of the long-term to short-term to major definite purpose goal implementation strategy. When we started working together, Patricia was working as a supermarket cashier and trying to earn enough money to launch her career as a paralegal so that she could accomplish her goals of becoming financially self-reliant and enhancing her quality of life. After taxes, Patricia took home two thousand dollars per month.

She determined that she needed to save twenty-five hundred dollars for a more reliable car and two months of auto insurance (her car was unfixable and she was getting around by bus when she created this plan).

Patricia had recently ended an abusive relationship, and her ex-boyfriend vindictively kept all of her belongings—including her clothes—which he later destroyed. Although she had won a judgment against him in court, it was nearly impossible to get him to re-pay her. He was unstable, and moved from friend's couch to friend's couch.

Patricia also needed to pass a test to obtain a specialized certification that would allow her to work for a certain type of law firm (the kind of law firm that she wanted to prospect for employment). The cost of the test, together with a test preparation course, was four hundred dollars. She also needed professional attire that she budgeted at six hundred dollars to start. All totaled, Patricia needed thirty-five hundred dollars.

She decided that since her main job at the supermarket was in the morning, she could work a second job in the evening for a period of time—long enough to earn what she needed to move to the next level and obtain her ultimate objective.

She took a second job working an average of twenty hours per week, at eleven dollars per hour. After taxes, she was able to clear roughly six hundred dollars per month of additional income. In less than six months, Patricia achieved her major definite purpose and short-term goals, and was well on her way towards achieving her long-term goals.

Since that time, Patricia has started working in the career of her dreams (with great benefits!) and has never been happier. She works forty hours per week again, and makes more money than in her two prior jobs combined.

She was recently able to obtain a low interest loan on a reasonably priced shiny new car that she can easily afford. She is empowered, dating, looks great in her new wardrobe, and lives in a new apartment. The future looks bright for Patricia, not just because of her new circumstances, but because of what she learned about herself (and the power of goals!) along the way.

As for the former boyfriend, he tried to contact her on a couple of occasions to see if she would consider being together again. The old Patricia might have said "yes." Now, she has changed phone numbers and would not go back to him for anything. Why would she? These days she has plenty of young hot-shot attorneys checking her out!

By embracing her goals and dreams, Patricia's cognitive world expanded. She soon discovered a whole new mind-set full of untapped possibilities. Due to goals, her confusion, depression, and instability disappeared, and she became anchored and fueled by goal-setting. Her plan to improve her life worked. It can work for you too!

Did you correctly identify the various stages of the goal-setting and implementation process?

Answers: 1.The obtainment of a second job that would provide enough money to move to the next steps ($3,500. total) represented Patricia's Major Definite Purpose (MDP); 2. Acquiring reliable transportation and car insurance, taking a test preparation course, passing her certification exam, purchasing new professional attire, and maintaining an enduring commitment to remain free from her former abusive boyfriend represent Patricia's short-term goals (STG); and 3. Landing a job with a desired firm, obtaining job benefits with a reasonable work load (40 hours per week) and good pay, obtaining an ever newer and more reliable car, and moving into a comfortable apartment represent her long-term goals (LTG) of becoming financially self-reliant and enhancing her quality of life.

In summary, Patricia absolutely crushed her goals! She is to be commended for her determination, focus, and success.

Goals and Your Attention Activating System

Clearly defined, time-bound goals prompt your reticular cortex (attention activating system) to engage, which helps you focus and attract into your life the circumstances and resources necessary to accomplish your objectives. As Patricia's story so clearly illustrates, it is important to combine action, hard work, and lots of inward desire when striving towards your objective(s).

Consider transferring (re-write, print, or photo copy) your top ten goals from your journal or organizer onto three-by-five index cards, and then tuck them into your purse or wallet. You may recall that in a previous session (Eight, Vision) we reviewed the importance of duration, frequency, intensity, and vividness within the context of imbedding your goals deeply into your mind. Carrying your goals with you permits instant access, so that you can review them often, even at a moment's notice.

My Personal Method

I maintain my work from the clarifying exercises, together with my goals lists (*Wish List* and *Blueprint for Life Success*), clearly laid out in a binder that I keep in my office at home. I have my top ten goals (LTG, STG, and MDP) organized (I do recommend that your index card remain focused on your top ten to fifteen goals, as more than that diminishes your ability to focus and complete a thorough review) on three index cards that I keep in my wallet at all times. Anyone who knows me well can testify to this fact. While I do not review my goals with just anyone (they are personal), I do keep them for my personal review (twice per day), and as a demonstration to my clients, family, and friends of just how serious I am about this powerful process. While my long-term goals do not change (except for relatively minor details), my short-term goals are more fluid, in that, as I accomplish various short-term objectives, new ones take their place. My major definite purpose changes in accordance with new (sometimes daily) challenges that must be met en route to accomplishing my life goals.

In addition to the aforementioned, in my organizer you would also see a running *Creative Ideas List* on which I write new ideas as they come to me. I then incorporate these into various aspects of my life and goals as applicable. For instance, an idea for a group coaching format, book, or seminar may strike me at any time; so I would jot this down on the list, and then review it as part of my morning routine; keeping and incorporating what seems like a good idea; and tossing it aside if I determine that it is not something I wish to implement after all.

Also, in my binder you would see a *Daily Virtues Practice Log*, wherein I track my daily performance on twelve key character, lifestyle, and personality virtues that I am endeavoring to strengthen, such as, balancing my personal and professional life more effectively; developing deeper levels of compassion, generosity, and humility; enhancing my ability to remember the names of people; and becoming a better listener, etc. (Please see Session Twelve, Courage for more on virtue development).

Finally, you would see a *Key Skills and Professional Development Survey* in which I routinely track my personal development in the areas of public speaking; teaching; writing; authenticity when engaged in one-on-one verbal communication; business finance management; time management; and the like. I exercise ten at the present moment.

Developing a Daily Routine

Each weekday morning, I start with exercise (even if it is something as simple as a good brisk walk); personal spiritual devotions (prayer for my family and clients, wherein I focus on their needs); a review of my life's goals (LTG, STG, and MDP); an exercise in present realization; a daily schedule review; a few moments of meditation on the characteristics, qualities, and skills outlined in the Daily Virtues Practice Log and Key Skills and Professional Development Survey (I review progress at the end of the day); and then I recite my positive affirmations while I get ready . . . starting with a good breakfast. All totaled, my morning preparation (including exercise, breakfast, and getting ready) takes two hours from start to finish.

As a single father of two, when my children are with me (as they often are), I simply get up earlier, get them ready, and build this morning routine around their needs and my work for that particular day. It all gets done, even if it means starting work a little bit later.

I find these disciplines so important, that while I love what I do for a living and would like very much to get started working by seven a.m., my standard schedule is to start work at nine a.m., to allow sufficient time for this preparation to occur. As a result, I find the time during the work day is much better spent, and I typically feel satisfied that I have accomplished what was most needed by the time I close my computer and leave the office at 6:30, 7, or 8pm. I do not work weekends unless I have a speaking engagement, a coaching group or class, or to meet a special client need.

Writing Down and Reviewing Your Goals

Writing down your goals and reviewing them often (in the morning, again at night some time before bed, and during the day whenever you have a few spare moments) impresses them into your subconscious mind. This, of course, activates your reticular cortex and amplifies the law of attraction. Also, it is energizing to review your goals and assists with maintaining a positive attitude, and a powerful, can-do mind-set.

Imagine your goals as a reality. See yourself at the goal, enjoying the goal, having achieved the goal. As you do this, you will see positive changes begin to take place, and an increased confidence that your goals are indeed achievable.

Even if your routine is quite simple, such as, a morning goals review, positive affirmations, and daily action steps towards achieving the things that you have identified as most important in your life, then you will be miles ahead of eighty to ninety percent of the population, and well on your way towards a richer, more prosperous, and enjoyable life.

Session Recap

Now would be a good time to complete the following:

1. Clarify what it is you want by using the clarifying and mind-expanding questions provided, e.g. *Magic Pill* and *Life's Last Days*

2. Create your *One Page Miracle for the Soul* (see Part One sample) and *Wish List*

3. Ask yourself, *"What Do I Most Enjoy Doing?"*

4. Identify and list, in personal, positive, and present tense, and using brief sentences, your long-term goals (what you truly want for your life), the steps necessary to get there (short-term goals), and the one, two, or three things that you first need to accomplish in order to accelerate the accomplishment of your goals expeditiously.

5. Keep your goals and action steps organized in a binder or notebook so that you can review them daily and make modifications as needed.

6. Create a list of your top ten goals, and place them in your wallet or purse for review whenever you get a few spare moments.

7. Develop a daily routine similar to the one that I've outlined above. *I am not Superman, and you do not have to be either. While I feel it is essential to remain faithful to your routine in order to obtain maximum benefit, the reality is that things come up, and we sometimes get sidetracked. Just do the best you can!*

8. Remember to develop your blueprint with the Life Balance chart handy to ensure that you carefully consider all of the important areas of your life and include them in your life success strategy.

So get moving! Identify what it is you want, create your life success goals blueprint, and then work on your goals every single day!

Session Eleven

Attitude

Say you are well, or all is well with you, and God shall hear your words and make them come true.

-Ella Wheeler Wilcox

It is highly symbolic that this session on Attitude just so happens to come at the very center (the heart) of Part Two. It was not intentionally planned this way. However, appropriate.

A powerful foundation for this entire book lies in the reality that "in almost everything, there is a grain of equal or greater opportunity." It takes a mental shift (producing serious cognitive cleansing!), and to some degree, a spiritual shift—faith, to grasp and apply this reality in day-to-day life. However, once you have made this shift, your life will likely never be the same.

Why will your life likely never be the same once you make this shift? Because you will have come to recognize that virtually everything that happens in your life can be utilized towards positive ends—if you have eyes to see.

All Things Work Together for Good

One of my favorite scripture passages (Romans, Chapter 8:28) says, "All things work together for good to those who love God, and are called according to His purpose." These words were preached from the Apostle Paul to the Romans.

This passage reminds us that although we may not always understand the reasons for suffering and pain, nevertheless, the closer our heart remains to God, the more faith we secure that everything will work out for good in the end.

Momentously, the more faith we secure, the more we can trust, and the more we can trust, the more we can hold securely to His promises. God's promises serve to steady our steps and anchor our decisions—despite our often all too limited human understanding.

The Pruning Process

Realizing that God is in the business of creating rose gardens of our lives, and therefore, has a purpose—that of fostering greater intimacy with Him, deepening our love, and pruning our character for usefulness—in allowing difficulties, also helps us better understand life's pain and struggles.

Through a faith informed positive attitude, we can more readily experience the fragrant aroma emanating from our present struggles, urging us to trust in the All Capable One who has promised to never leave or forsake us. This perspective results in greater joy, peace, and personal power.

Every branch that bears fruit, He [God] prunes it, that it may bear more fruit.
-John 15:2

Romans 8:28 and the pruning process metaphor in scripture refer primarily to spiritually-derived attitudinal factors, since they presuppose an understanding of God's omnipotence and benevolence in managing the affairs of His people. However, the following illustrations refer mainly to inwardly-derived attitudinal factors, emanating from personal decisions representing one's manner of response to life's difficulty. Hence the following question: when life hands you lemons, will you make lemonade, or put on a sour face?

A person of personal power, whom I have really come to admire, is former United States Secretary of State, Condoleezza Rice.

Attitude Trumps Bigotry

In an interview aired on NPR, October 13, 2010, Dr. Condoleezza Rice discussed her family life as a young African American residing in Alabama.

I was so impressed by the fact that, though Dr. Rice acknowledged the reality of racism in her community, she and the members of her family refused to be victims of it. Intrigued by the interview, I pulled my car over, and between bites of a ham and egg bagel sandwich and sips of morning coffee, began taking notes.

It became immediately evident to me that Dr. Rice's father was anything but a victim. In fact, he was a fighter!

She tells a story about the time she and her family went to see Santa Claus, and her father said, "If Santa Claus is going to treat you differently, and hold you at a distance . . ." (Her father perceived that the black kids were being held at a further distance from Santa's body and lap than the white kids) ". . . then I will expose Santa Claus for who he is, a 'cracker,' and I will rip the heck out of him." This fighting spirit did not end with her father.

Her family, together with her community, determined that in order to level the playing field, they would need to be educated and speak well. So, taking matters into their own hands, they worked hard to acquire the skills, qualities, and characteristics necessary for success in twentieth century America.

While remaining well aware of the dangers of living in Alabama at that time, Dr. Rice's family maintained a mentality of do-it-ive-ness, possibility thinking, inner-strength, and self-determination, as opposed to cowering in fear and creating excuses for why they could not excel.

As the former United States Secretary of State, and an accomplished public speaker and professor, Dr. Rice has obviously risen to great heights. She and her family have provided a shining example of what it means to triumph over adversity through the power of exercising a positive attitude.

She Did Not Push Back!

Another touching story, drawn from the life of someone who recently experienced tragedy, exemplifies the kind of attitude to which this book now turns attention. It's the story of twenty-four year old college graduate, Rachelle Friedman. You may recall seeing the story in the press. I became aware of it through a Today Show interview that I saw via the internet, dated November 22, 2010.

According to the interview and documentary, Rachelle was just weeks away from what by nearly all accounts promised to be a perfect wedding, to the "perfect fiancé," when she (at her own bachelorette party) was pushed into the pool by a prank while horsing around. What started as a celebration with some of her closest friends suddenly became tragic.

In a freak accident, the push caused Rachelle to hit her head in the pool. She became paralyzed, sustaining a C-6 spinal cord injury. The injury destroyed her ability to feel below her collar bone.

However, her spirit remains intact!

After a stay in Intensive Care and three months in the hospital, as of the writing of this book, Rachelle continues to go to outpatient therapy, and despite being told that she will never be able to walk again, has been able to regain the use of her arms, and is working hard to regain other lost functions.

A portion of her success she attributes to the loving support of family, friends, and of course, her fiancé (school teacher Chris Chapman). Rachel and Chris stated that they fully intend on going through with the wedding at a future, yet to be determined date.

When asked about harboring resentment, Rachelle (who refuses to reveal the name of the friend who pushed her in the pool) stated, "blaming her would be ridiculous," maintaining that "It was a freak accident" and could happen to anyone.

When asked about the role of attitude in her recovery and positive disposition toward the future, Rachelle stated, "Almost all of it is attitude." She continues, "If you are not willing to do the work to get better, you won't. . . . I just worked really hard to do as much as I could, as fast as I could. . . . Think about what you can do, not what you can't do."

Obviously, this would be a tragic incident for anyone, especially for a soon-to-be bride. Yet, this story portrays so much about attitude, self-determination, forgiveness, courage, self-discipline, and persistence, that it serves as a classic example of what this session is intended to convey.

Attitude Determines Altitude.

-Captain Shannon L. Jipsen

Attitude: A Determining Factor

The ability to reframe life's difficulties in order to turn tragedy into triumph all begins with a positive state of mind. Virtually every noteworthy individual who has ever walked the face of the earth became successful by cultivating a positive and constructive attitude. In fact, countless books, lectures, and sermons have identified this virtue, time and again, as perhaps the most essential component to life success.

The longer I live the more I realize the impact of attitude on life. Attitude, to me, is more important than facts. It is more important than the past, than education, than money, than circumstances, than failures, than successes, than what other people think or say or do. It is more important than appearance, giftedness, or skill. It will make or break a company . . . a church . . . a home.

-Chuck Swindoll

Adversity Strengthens Character

While every session in this book is important, this session, perhaps above all others, is crucial to your success. It is the session upon which all of the other sessions rest. In fact, the preeminent role of attitude in success has been esteemed as such by virtually all great philosophers, playwrights, poets, and leaders throughout the centuries. Here are a few examples.

A man without a smiling face must not open a shop.

-Chinese Proverb

Events will take their course, it is no good of being angry at them; he is happiest who wisely turns them to the best account.

-Euripides

I became acquainted with those martyrs whose behavior in camp, who's suffering and death, bore witness to the fact that the last inner freedom cannot be lost. . . . Everything can be taken from a man but one thing; the last of the human freedoms to choose one's attitude in any given set of circumstances, to choose one's own way. . . . Most men in a concentration camp believed that the real opportunities of life had passed. Yet, in reality, there was an opportunity and a challenge. One could make a victory of those circumstances, turning life in to an inner triumph, or one could ignore the challenge and simply vegetate, as did a majority of the prisoners.

-Viktor Frankl, neuroscientist, psychiatrist, Holocaust survivor

There is nothing either good or bad, but thinking makes it so.

-William Shakespeare

Meet Attitude's Cousin, Reframe

Reframing can be described as an attitudinal technique wherein one chooses to interpret a situation, event, or circumstance in a positive and constructive light. I first learned of reframing as a graduate student working towards a master's degree in counseling, and have used it ever since. It is an incredibly powerful tool both for work with clients, as well as having application to one's personal life.

Many people have come to realize that their perception of something will often determine the end result, and that how they frame life's events will either empower or restrict them. I find this to be so true.

A simple example of a reframe is when you determine that the delay in the line at the grocery store is not the end of the world, but rather, an opportunity to practice the virtues of patience and generosity by deciding you are going to buy groceries for the struggling parent who is in line with four kids.

A Lawyer's Shining Moment

A more elaborate example of reframing can be drawn from a lawyer client of mine (we'll call him, "John") who failed to make Partner at a firm for whom he had poured blood, sweat, and tears for over twelve years. He was so upset that he impulsively left the firm and awoke the next day (two months before Christmas!) to find himself unemployed.

John had a lovely wife (who had supported him through law school) and three children (ages four, eight, and thirteen) to feed, and a mortgage and bills totaling over nine thousand dollars in monthly payments. He had burned his bridge with the firm so badly, that returning was simply not an option.

He and I sought for ways that he could get back on his feet and leverage this situation to not only secure his survival, but also to work powerfully in his favor. We created an inventory of his assets and strengths (financial, personal, and professional) and we quickly developed a game plan for success.

A significant part of rallying for success, for John, involved a major attitude check. When he began to realize that his attitude (he was often negative—a trait he recalls inheriting from his father) contributed to his inability to make Partner, he determined to begin seeing things in a more positive light. Although it took some time, clear evidence of a major attitude shift began to emerge. His attitude transformation became so pervasive that it spilled over onto his wife and three children.

John went from being desperate about his situation to brimming with life and optimism. About eight weeks into coaching, just before the New Year, he received an offer to join a firm that he had respected and admired for some time. He recalls, "It wasn't until I became desperate after losing my job that I realized just how much I was missing (both personally and

139

professionally) by being so negative all the time. I had spent a better part of my adult life enduring negativity in my soul, and being a real downer for those closest to me." He began to see how his negative attitude had impacted virtually all areas of his life, and how having a positive attitude could take him farther than he had ever thought possible. When John contacted me two years later, he was enjoying his experience at the firm, loving life, and full of positive energy and enthusiasm.

The best part is I didn't even have to provide the reframe for this one. John provided the reframe himself. His last words to me were, "If I hadn't lost my job, none of this would have been possible. Next to my wife and kids, losing my job was probably the best thing to ever happen to me." I agreed. This is a prime example of reframing a potentially bad situation into a learning and growing opportunity.

I have seen time and again the crucial role that attitude plays in determining the quality of one's life by influencing the course of a person's destiny. Attitude, according to the late, great, Coach John Wooden, is ever important, as, "Things turn out best for the people who make the best of the way things turn out."

In our day-to-day lives we are sure to experience obstacles and setbacks. However, with a positive attitude and diligent effort things are bound to work out well.

Locus of Control—What Describes You?

Years ago, as a counselor trainee, I became aware of a set of terms which helped me to better organize and express what I thought I had already observed in peoples' personalities with regards to their dispositions towards life. The terms are *internal locus of control* and *external locus of control*, meaning that an individual is a passive responder, *external*, or a powerful shaper, *internal*, of the events and circumstances surrounding his or her life.

Locus of control refers to one's beliefs and perceptions about the underlying main causes of events in his or her life, i.e., one's attitude, behavior, and destiny are either guided by fate, luck, and a variety of external forces—what happens *to* them, or one's attitude, behavior, and destiny are controlled by personal decisions and actions—what he or she *makes* happen.

This is not to say that being externally set is altogether a liability. For instance, people with this disposition have a tendency to be a bit more relaxed, easy-going, and happy-go-lucky in certain situations. However, a potentially serious drawback to maintaining this disposition lies in the tendency to be passive, as opposed to active, in the shaping of one's life. And, when circumstances don't happen to be good (which, as we know, they often are not!), they lack the internal drive necessary to shift the tide in order to make things better, and therefore, are more prone to fall victims of circumstance—potentially leading to a condition known as *learned helplessness*, or depression.

Individuals with a personality disposition towards that of internal locus of control refuse to be a victim. Instead, they view life's circumstances as something they must master internally, as representing opportunities for personal growth. These people are powerful, because, virtually everything that happens to them is viewed as an opportunity to learn, grow, and affect a better outcome. Therefore, they perceive that life's circumstances can potentially almost always work out in their favor—with proper planning and focused effort.

Research shows that people higher up in organizational structures tend to be more internal (Mamlin, Harris, & Case, 2001), and they tend to be more achievement oriented and obtain better paying jobs. Additionally, individuals with an internal locus of control tend to maintain an increased sense of psychological well-being and are much more adept to living in the social world. Finally, it is important to point out that research in psychology seems to support the notion that locus of control is not so much genetic, as it is learned and environmentally shaped. This lends further support to the notion of *choice* as discussed in Part One, Session Three.

Meet Susan

A few years ago, I had a client come to see me. Her name is Susan. Susan had just lost one of her breasts to cancer, and wanted to learn to move forward with her life in a positive way, but she was having difficulty managing this tremendous loss. As an unusually attractive woman in her late-thirties, Susan had grown accustomed to basing her identity on her physical beauty and curvaceous figure. Now, for the first time in her life, she was forced to look within, and she did not like what she saw.

Susan had fallen into the trap, like so many women in our culture today, of defining her life merely by her external appearance. She recalls, "I lived for so many years depending on my looks. It defined me. I was able to get whatever I wanted, whenever I wanted it, and however I wanted it. Other than finishing a couple years of college, I did not cultivate any marketable job skills, and never really had to hear the word, 'No.' I took so much for granted. I couldn't imagine that life could change on a dime. In the midst of this illness, my boyfriend of five years broke up with me, my finances became a wreck, and many of my friends have abandoned me. Now I am left with nothing!"

Susan now had to rebuild her life on a new paradigm. Together with grief work, this became the central purpose of our counseling sessions.

For a period of eight months, we worked together and she was able to re-discover inner resources that lay dormant. She was determined to re-define herself, not on the basis of appearance alone, but on the basis of the whole of life. She made the transition herself. Oh sure, I assisted, but she is the one who had to draw on her inner resources in order to make progress. It was up to her to make the attitude adjustment necessary to see her situation in a positive light, and, drawing on her inner resources, determine to be a success.

During the eight months that we worked together, we were able to do an inventory of her skills, gifts, and talents. Based on that information, she enrolled in college with a desire to become a nurse. She also began challenging previously held beliefs about her love life and how she defined both her value and role as a woman.

In time, a whole new world opened-up for her, because she *chose* to interpret this event in her life as an opportunity, as opposed to a tragedy. As the saying goes, "When life hands you lemons, make lemonade."

A while back Susan contacted me. She is making good progress in nursing school, and has met a great guy who she says, "loves me for me."

They are engaged to be married in December of 2011. She is excited about her future and has a passion for helping people. In her role as a nurse, she will have ample opportunity to do just that!

A Grain of Equal or Greater Opportunity

The person with an internal locus of control believes that life's challenges are filled with opportunity, and they act accordingly.

The mindset of success must rest on the premise which says, "no matter what happens to me, or around me, I am committed to grasping the positive in any situation, to the best extent that I am capable. I am going to choose the outcomes of my life by interpreting life's circumstances, not as a victim, but as an active free-agent in determining the outcomes of my life, and by seeing the opportunity, lesson, and glimmer of possibility in virtually everything."

This kind of attitude presupposes that one's life is oriented towards personal growth and is not defined by superficial things, but rather, by esteeming and valuing the timeless characteristics of spirituality—love, meaning, and purpose.

Nothing can stop the man with the right mental attitude from achieving his goal; nothing on earth can help the man with the wrong mental attitude.

-Thomas Jefferson

Session Twelve

Courage

Of all the attributes of mankind, the most important is courage because that's the one that guarantees all the others.

-Winston Churchill

Often when discussing courage, we think of a soldier on the field of battle, or firefighters who rushed into the burning twin towers, or images of Martin Luther King, Jr. marching on Washington D.C. where he delivered his now famous, "I Have A Dream" speech. Certainly, these are all fitting examples of courage—the first two of physical courage, and the last, moral courage—the courage of conviction (Miller, 2005).

For centuries, philosophers have debated the true meaning of courage, attributing various characteristics, such as bravery, conviction, and virtue, depending on the circumstances surrounding a particular personality or event. However, for our purposes, rather than critically analyze the philosophical nuances of courage, we will blend commonly conceded elements in hopes of obtaining a better understanding of how this essential attribute plays a crucial role in determining life success.

Defining Courage

Drawing from the scenarios presented above, we would likely agree that courage involves, at minimum, bravery and the ability to withstand discomfort, fear, pain, danger, or uncertainty. However, moral courage can be differentiated from physical courage, in that, it often occurs without a feeling of accomplishment, reward, or acknowledgement, and is revealed in more common, uncelebrated, day-to-day experiences and decisions in which one holds true to his or her convictions despite difficulty (Miller, 2005).

This often obscure form of courage has always fascinated me. Paradoxically, while being the least mentioned, it is arguably the most pervasive prerequisite to personal success.

In our modern way of life, most of us will never enter a burning building, or engage in a gun battle. However, on a daily basis we all face difficult life decisions that must be made, decisions that challenge both our courage and convictions.

In light of these observations, courage defined as *moral courage, holding true to ones convictions*, or *someone willing to step outside of his or her comfort zone and take risks* ("leaps of faith") in order to improve his or her life, or expand his or her influence in the world, will be of primary focus in this session.

The ultimate measure of a man is not where he stands in moments of comfort and convenience, but where he stands at times of challenge and controversy.

-Martin Luther King, Jr.

Self as the Greatest Enemy

Philosopher Immanuel Kant pointed out long ago that people's ideals sometimes conflict with their desires. Therefore, according to Kant, the conquest of self represents one of the more intense of human struggles. Perhaps this helps explain why inconsistency in following one's values often emerges as a contributing factor to failure in a person's life.

The willingness to deny gratification of undesirable or otherwise self-destructive behavior in order to realize a richer outcome has all but disappeared in a morally and spiritually pluralistic culture. Increasingly, right and wrong have become difficult to define, and character is too often pawned as a diminishing commodity. Francis J. Beckwith and

Gregory Koukl insightfully refer to this as "Relativism: Feet Firmly Planted in Mid-Air" (1998).

Herein lies an oft-overlooked and even surprising definition of courage—a person's willingness to stay the course amidst adversity, especially when everyone else is doing something contrary.

Having determined that in our day-to-day lives the virtues of courage and conviction are important preludes to life success, it might be helpful to consider a couple of familiar individuals who embraced a similar notion, and with outstanding results.

George Washington and Success Virtues

George Washington, our nation's first President and an American Founding Father, was born of humble circumstances. As a young boy, at the age of fourteen, he had a natural disposition towards propriety—to such a degree, that he copied and memorized one hundred and ten rules for elegant deportment from a work created by Jesuits in the 16th century, which served as a guide for "young gentleman of quality."

We are told that, in large part through the practice of such virtues, George Washington later became known as one of the most respected leaders of history. He was also regarded as one of the most gentlemanly men, and a decisive and courageous leader with a deep commitment to justice, leadership, and success. His philosophical insights fortified his ability to earn the admiration and respect of those under his charge, which was crucial to American progress at an extraordinarily critical time in our nation's history.

George Washington, together with many other great men and women of courage and conviction, served as a catalyst for what would eventually result in freedom from British tyranny, and the founding of the greatest nation in world history.

Benjamin Franklin and a Key Virtues List

Benjamin Franklin, American publisher and statesman, recognized that he would need to develop certain personality characteristics, key virtues if you will, if he was to excel in his business and political life in early American society. Among the thirteen virtues in all (Franklin, 1732) he lists the *personal virtues* of temperance, moderation, and industry, etc.; under *social virtues* he lists sincerity, justice, and humility, etc.

History tells us that he kept a notebook and daily virtues progress chart with him for most of his life (much like the one discussed in Session Ten).

It is important to bear in mind that Benjamin Franklin did not always succeed, but sometimes strayed from his personal and social objectives. However, at least he was trying, and likely progressed much further in his life as a result.

What about You?

Could it be that part of your life recovery represents a return to the "basics and fundamentals"—to quote the late Coach John Wooden, *again*—of practicing the virtues that you know deep down to be right?

Courage and Leaps of Faith

The second definition of courage, as mentioned above, describes someone willing to step outside of his or her comfort zone and take risks—"leaps of faith"—in order to improve his or her life, or expand his or her influence in the world.

You have likely heard the American proverb, "Nothing ventured, nothing gained." A person might begin to wonder if this phrase was coined by the first American settlers. When you consider the treacherous waters the early settlers crossed in hopes of securing a better life—many of them simply did not make it—you realize just how big a leap of faith their journey really was. And although many lives were lost in the settling of this nation, those who courageously escaped Europe in search of freedom eventually found that for which they searched, and the world has never since been the same.

The very substance of the ambitious is merely the shadow of a dream.

-William Shakespeare

We only have one life to live. We must get real about what it is that we truly want. Might I even be so bold as to assert that it is time for us to quit playing games, and to begin imagining ourselves standing at the end-zone of life, asking these three crucial questions: "Who am I?" "What do I want to do with my life?" And "Who do I really want to be?"

Courage bridges the chasm between safety, boredom, and mediocrity on one hand, and risk, liveliness, and greatness on the other.

How is Virtue Developed?

Answer: Practice. Refer to the *Key Virtues List* that you've created. And Peer Support (spending time with eagles, not vultures).

By surrounding yourself with others willing to hold up your faltering arms when you grow weary—people who inspire, encourage, and cheer you onward—who will remind you of the strengths they see in you, you will develop virtue.

Surround Yourself with Eagles

As mentioned earlier, expect adversity when you step forth to accomplish something great. Some friends and family will become uncomfortable, even jealous of your success, and may seek to hold you back. Herein is manifest the all too familiar dynamic of homeostasis—*same* or *comfortable state*—when others want you to remain as they are, for fear of being left behind.

It will take courage to forge ahead towards your goals. By linking up with like-minded people striving for similar things, you are far more likely to move ahead much farther, much faster.

It is lonely at the top. Hang around with can-do people.

-Coach Mark Thomas

Step Out

There is nothing quite like stepping into your destiny by proceeding in the face of fear. You wake up one day to realize that what used to haunt you has been laid to rest. By facing your fears, you become their master, and your fears become familiar, conquered ground.

Ask Yourself

Have you ever asked yourself the following questions?

-What virtues will I need to cultivate in order to accomplish my life's objectives?

-What leaps of faith have I been avoiding?

-Do I welcome the call to step-out and begin really living?

-What am I prepared to do with this urging in my life right now?

In Conclusion

Every great venture requires courage, because venturing into unchartered territory means being confronted with circumstances that will test your character and convictions, and force you to confront your fears. But don't worry. Because when this occurs you will feel truly *alive*!

In fact, along the journey you may question your own sanity in pursuing your objectives. You will likely reason, "Others aren't doing this!" and then ask yourself, "Can I make it?" or "What if I don't make it?" However, you will likely gain courage by focusing on your goals, and recalling the consequences of remaining in that predictable and unfulfilling place where you were before setting out.

Remember, "No guts—No glory!"

SESSION THIRTEEN

DISCIPLINE

Life's a continuous business, and so is success, and requires continuous effort.

–Margaret Thatcher, former Prime Minister of Great Britain

The Role of Discipline in Success

In my practice, I use an initial intake questionnaire that asks, "Do you base decisions on your feelings?" and a majority of the people who come to see me answer "Yes" to this question. The very next question asks, "How is this working for you?" The typical response to this question is, "Not well."

A key aspect of discipline is the ability to do what we have to do, when it has to get done, regardless of our feelings.

Earlier we discussed cognition. Then we discussed ways to bypass negative emotions by establishing a goals blueprint that will keep you excited, anchored, and positive about your day-to-day life.

Discipline will come easier when you are excited about your journey. Much the same as it would be easier to get up on Monday morning to go and pick up a ten million dollar lottery check than it would be to go to work at a job that you do not enjoy.

Disciplining Your Mind

I am right brained by nature. I am a creative dreamer. That means, I have had to work really hard to develop the practical, *just do it* side of my personality. I use to follow my feelings, which equated to increasing difficulty in my life.

I have had to discipline myself over the years to follow good judgment, and to listen to my feelings constructively, but not let them rule my decisions. Developing this discipline has worked for me. It can work for you, too!

With discipline and goal setting, the feelings factor (that of being ruled by feelings) all but leaves the equation, as decisions are diverted more into the executive area of the brain, and feelings become a less dominant part of the equation. Therefore, it would be accurate to say that goals are "anchoring." Herein is New Mind Synergy (NMS = CG2) at work in a profound way.

Powerfully, a person who bases decisions on their goals is able to more readily bypass unconstructive thoughts and feelings, and is less subject to the cognitive roots of failure that we discussed in Part One. The result is that greater balance is restored to one's thought life. By emphasizing this in my practice, my clients seem to make more progress than before, oftentimes more quickly.

Shifts in Our Culture

In a culture with diminishing boundaries around personal behavior, feelings run-amok. Where there are limited boundaries, feelings become both the informer and interpreter of life events. This leads to a roller-coaster ride of unintended consequences.

I would be willing to bet that my survey question, "Do you base decisions on your feelings?" would have been answered far differently, for a majority of people, three, four, or five decades ago, at a time when moral absolutes and principles for living were often celebrated and reinforced. That is why my coaching programs also include the development of personal virtues, often reinforced within a small group setting.

Failure Rests in the Seemingly Little Things

Failure often occurs as a result of the things we fail to do. It could therefore be said that success is in the details. Victory goes to the one willing to work that much harder, stay in there that much longer, and keep trying until they get it right.

Oftentimes, when I do not feel like doing something, but I do it because I know it has to be done, when it has to be done, whether I like it or not, then I notice that things usually turn out really well for that day.

It is almost as if the greatest blessing is reserved for those days when it is the hardest to cooperate, but I do so anyway, because I know I must in order to achieve my objectives. Success pitches its tent within the valley of discipline.

Delaying Gratification

The ability to delay gratification is a lost art in our "serve me now" culture. This tendency squashes personal power.

Stanford University psychology researcher Walter Mischel conducted a study that began in the 1960s. In the study, children at the Bing Nursery School (located on the campus of Stanford University) were given an opportunity to eat a marshmallow right away, or wait fifteen or twenty minutes and receive two marshmallows.

According to the study, approximately one third of the children grabbed the marshmallow right away, a third waited several minutes before grabbing it, and the rest were able to wait the entire duration, and receive both of the marshmallows.

This study demonstrates a possible correlation between the ability to delay gratification and life success on a number of different fronts. Years later when the children graduated from high school the differences between the two groups were significant: the children who resisted the temptation were more positive, self motivated, and able to remain strong in the face of adversity toward the accomplishment of their life's goals. They had habits consistent with success, resulting in happier marriages, vocational satisfaction, financial stability, physical health, and higher levels of life satisfaction.

Those who gobbled-up the marshmallows were more troubled, hard-headed, indecisive, self-focused, mistrustful, less confident, and still not able to effectively delay gratification. Additionally, they were more easily distracted by stimuli that diverted attention away from their goals and objectives. These characteristics seemed to manifest diminished career satisfaction, financial instability, decreased marital contentment, poor physical health, and an overall diminished quality of life.

Walter Mischel asserts (after hundreds of hours of observation) that having creative ways to divert attention away from the object of temptation, and toward a more worthwhile goal, is crucial to success (Lehrer, 2009).

Many people don't succeed because they aren't willing to pay the price, to practice self-discipline, or to sacrifice en route to a higher goal or objective. They say they want success, but their actions are incongruent with their expressed objectives.

I believe this dissonance results from lack of clarity regarding what an individual truly wants for his or her life. Generally speaking, when people speak of wanting something, they oftentimes are merely expressing a dream or a wish, as opposed to a carefully analyzed (weighing the pro's and con's of the variables involved) life course.

This premise is consistent with Mischel's observations about the successful temptation resister, insofar as the power to resist lies in one's ability to distract him or herself by focusing away from the short-term reward, and onto something better, albeit future.

Two things, and two things only. Know exactly what you want, determine the price you will have to pay to get it, and then get busy paying that price.

-H.L. hunt, oil billionaire

Success: Many Years in the Making

Sometimes successful people appear on the scene suddenly, as if from nowhere. That is because, in most cases, the long, hard road to success remains undocumented. What the public sees is the sudden surge, the "big break" that actually resulted from years of hard work, careful planning, and personal sacrifice—all while very few people, if any, were watching. What may appear as a sudden rise to success may actually have been a decade or two in the making.

Research has demonstrated that the person who is willing to discipline him or herself until they obtain their ultimate objective(s) become happier people in the long run. Even the years they spend struggling at their craft, before the "big break," are years well lived—happiness is in the journey. Yes, it is these who will likely never have to say, "Would have," "Should have," or "Could have" because they will know, firsthand, what it is like to truly be alive.

Know prudent, cautious self-control is wisdom's root.

-Robert Burns

Session Fourteen

Persistence

Be of good cheer. Do not think of today's failures, but of the success that may come tomorrow. You have set for yourself a difficult task, but you will succeed if you persevere; and you will find a joy in overcoming obstacles.

-Helen Keller

Always remember,

Goal
Enriched
Thoughts
Ultimately
Prevail

Failure happens, and no one is immune. In fact, it seems the higher a person reaches, the more he or she is bound to experience failure.

Some of the world's most wealthy and successful people have repeated a mantra time and again, whether by speech or written word, that goes something like this: "Failure forged the steel of character to make me who I am today!"

A compilation of quotes and life stories amplifies this principle for us as follows:

History has demonstrated that the most notable winners usually encounter the most heartbreaking obstacles before they triumph. They won because they refused to become discouraged by their defeat.

-B.C. Forbes, founder of Forbes Magazine

You just keep pushing. You just keep pushing. I made every mistake that could be made, but I just kept pushing.

-Rene McPherson (former president of the Dana Corporation)

Our greatest glory is not in never falling, but in rising every time we fall.

-Confucius

It is believed that Thomas Edison experienced failure perhaps more than any other mover and shaker of the 20th century. Maybe that is because he seemingly attempted more things than any other person. Nevertheless, building on his mistakes, and refusing to quit, he succeeded in more things than anyone else, and contributed to the advancement of American life in extraordinarily valuable ways.

A Coach's Example

Remember Coach Mark Thomas—the one who trained me in sales? He once told the story of how he used to sit over his cereal at the family breakfast table every morning before work, and give his empty hand (as if shaking sugar onto his cereal) a few shakes before eating. Of course, initially, his wife asked, "What are you doing?" To which he responded, "I am shaking rejection over my cereal, because I know that I am going to experience plenty of it today. . . . I am preparing myself in advance."

This is a man who, despite being among the top sales professionals in the country, routinely experienced rejection, and understood the value of preparing his attitude in preparation for each new day. By sticking to his plan and persevering through whatever failures came his way, he remained successful.

Pushing To the Front!

Orison Swett Marden, the writer of the timeless classic, *Pushing To The Front* (first published in 1894) understood the value of perseverance.

Dr. Marden was a studious young man who graduated from Boston University in 1871 with a degree in law, and then later from Harvard with an M.D., and LL. B. degrees (1881-1882 respectively).

Throughout the early days of his career, he became a hotel and resort owner, until financial reverses ended that career.

Around this time, Dr. Marden began to study the practices of America's greatest leaders, making notes along the way. He determined to write a book based on what he had learned from personal experience, as well as through influences such as Samuel Smiles, Oliver Wendell Holmes, Jr., and Ralph Waldo Emerson.

Dr. Marden became a strong believer that each person determines his or her destiny, not by chance or good fortune, but through personal willpower and persistent effort.

What makes Dr. Marden's philosophy so poignant is the fact that his parents died while he was a boy—his mother while he was age 3, and his father at age 7—and he and his sisters were shuffled from guardian to guardian, where they often worked as "hired help." He supported himself through his education, as there was no silver spoon in the waiting for young Orison.

However, adversity did not end there. After losing his original book manuscript, some 1500 pages and nearly two years in the making, in a house fire, Dr. Marden determined to persevere. Drawing on his inner-resources of desire, passion, and motivation, he decided to take up the work of writing his book, yet again, starting from scratch. It might even be aptly stated that this event (the fire) sparked an even greater mobilization of his internal drive, stronger than he had ever known heretofore.

Marden finally completed his manuscript, and it was published (800 plus pages) in 1894.

Pushing To The Front became a best selling American classic. It is hailed as one of the most influential books on business success ever written, and is credited as having influenced thousands of people towards greatness at a time when America desperately needed inspiration—as the great depression and two world wars would descend upon the nation in the succeeding four decades.

The books excerpt states, "It is doubtful whether any other book, outside of the Bible, has been the turning-point in more lives."

What if Dr. Marden had allowed the fire to ruin his dream of publishing what is now considered a great American classic? How differently would thousands, even millions, of lives have been lived? How very different might *your* life be today?

In celebrating these stories, we celebrate perseverance at its best.

The Persistence Test

There is often an especially difficult period of time just prior to any significant breakthrough. It is often referred to as "the persistence test." It's as if we are tested one last grueling time in order to prepare our hearts for what we are about to receive (clarity), strengthen our spiritual and psychological muscles to ensure that we can handle it (readiness), and to reserve a special blessing for our having had the faith to persevere (faith).

Passion Does Not Mean Easy

Being passionate about achieving a desired objective or developing a coveted skill or ability does not necessarily mean that we can take possession of it with ease. While the things for which we are passionate tend to come easier than, for instance, something for which we have no passion, we do well to realize that difficulty itself forms the catalyst for greatness. A task must be difficult if we are to engage all of the various elements of heart, soul, and spirit that make the attainment of an objective ultimately rewarding.

Where no sparks fly, there is no forging and shaping, and hence, no ultimate passion can truly exist. Therefore, we realize that being great at something we love often entails hard work.

Mindful of this, we come to expect and even embrace difficulty, rather than be caught off guard by it (referring once again to the king and builder illustrations in Part One, Session Two).

When we persevere despite difficulty, our skills and abilities have a chance to mature. Under the tutelage of adversity our task muscles grow, and so too does our capacity to receive in fuller measure that which we love. It is then that we become great, as set apart from those not willing to engage in the arduous process that greatness requires of its possessors.

That is why persistence is so very necessary—if for no other reason than to conquer the earthy elements of gravity, space, and time required to achieve mastery—at which point, an attribute, skill, or ability becomes second nature.

When something becomes second nature, it is then that our genius has a chance to emerge. Genius cannot emerge before mastery, because until mastery, our focus is on clumsily managing the issue or task itself, and not on the more creative, higher order elements thereof. But, once the task is automatic, we are home free—if we keep at it.

The best results happen when we do not feel like going any further, but do so anyway—this is where the richness lies. And it is persistence that brings such richness into our lives.

Kites rise against, not with the wind.

-Orison Swett Marden

Blueprinting Well
& Conclusion

Happiness is the state of consciousness which proceeds from the achievement of one's values.

-Ayn Rand

I can still recall attending my step-grandfather's funeral. It was held on a warm, sunny, late summer day in Orlando, Florida, September 16, 1994. His name was Herman C. Ray.

Grandfather Ray was a good man, a man of faith. He lived out his beliefs in a quiet, gentle, and consistent manner. Among other things, I recall that he always had time to tend to the needs of others—whether it was taking me to the beach during one of my breaks from high school, or sending a word of encouragement in the form of a carefully written letter to a family member who might be struggling with an issue in their life. Grandfather Ray was always prepared to lend a thoughtful, helping hand.

Upon reflecting, I am also struck by the effortlessness with which he lived his life. He seemed to balance his family, work, church, and personal life with precision. Perhaps that is why he was so available to serve others?

As a career minister, and then a chaplain at Orlando's Florida Hospital for a certain portion of his life, he remained devoted to the service and well-being of others. At his funeral, there was no shortage of people present to testify to the profound impact he had had on their life. I can still recall how deeply the stories impacted me. Moved in a powerful way, it's as if I was experiencing a sweet and abiding foretaste of heaven, and of God's love.

My senses were further awakened by an abundant array of plants, fragrant and colorful bouquets of flowers, a sprawling landscape of freshly cut grass, warm sunshine, and white, puffy clouds—prompting vivid memories of funerals I have attended that stood in stark contrast to this bitter-sweet anomaly. This was more a celebration of a life well-lived, than a ceremony for mourning.

I determined that day to leave a similar legacy—not merely for personal recognition, but for the sheer beauty of a life devoted to all that is right, all that is good, all that is love.

Since that day so many years ago, my life has not always traveled along a straight and narrow road. There have been a fair amount of twists and turns—and some of them quite painful—as well as some successes and triumphs.

However, the desire remains—perhaps stronger now than ever—to both live, and finish, well. In my estimation, there would be no sweeter destiny than to fulfill the vision that was captured that warm summer day, September 16, 1994.

The Finish Line of Life

Ultimately, all of us will stand at the finish line of life, where we will have only our choices, words, actions, and the testimony of others to serve as a reflection of our successes or failures. In light of this, it seems fitting to consider our life's blueprint carefully, and to blueprint well.

The Importance of Balance

Balance is a crucial element for life success. Without balance, we become one-sided, off-kilter, and therefore, unhealthy and ineffective.

I recall some years ago a pastor telling the story of a "poor" man in his congregation who had lost his wife and children. Oh! He was not poor monetarily! Nor did his wife and children die. In fact, quite the contrary was true. They were very much alive, just no longer living at home. He was poor because his life was imbalanced. He had spent all of his time amassing wealth, and in the process, had neglected the intimacy needs of his family.

Responding to an urgent plea by the poor man to "Please come quickly!", the pastor made his way to the home and up the long, winding driveway that lined the poor man's sprawling estate. As he reached the top of the hill, he gazed through the windshield of his car, where he could see the poor man—face in hands, his body convulsing with howling sobs—seated on the cold concrete circular driveway just outside the entrance of his home. Being aware of the family's troubles, it did not take long for the pastor to grasp both the nature and gravity of this visitation request.

Placing a gentle hand on the poor man's shoulder, the pastor listened and attempted to lend comfort and support. After nearly an hour of regretfully recounting all the many ways that he had not been there for his family, the poor man then admitted something profound. He said, "I would give everything I have for just an ounce of the peace that you have, Pastor!"

Being deeply impacted by the visit, as the pastor drove home that night, his mind was drawn to the ways in which he himself was not fully present for the members of his own family. He remembered basketball dates missed with his sons, baseball games that he was just too busy to attend, and a father and daughter dance that he missed while out of town attending an "important conference." He made the decision right there and then to make the priority shifts necessary to put "first-things-first" in his own family life. He later stated, "I have never regretted that decision."

Towards a Holistic Approach

Reflecting on the life balance chart provided in Session Ten, we come to realize that virtually every crucial area of our existence is addressed therein. Each of the six areas serves as important facets of our lives, and therefore, cannot be ignored.

From the story of the "poor" man, to the pastors own personal struggle with balance, we can see the tremendous importance of a holistic (all-inclusive) approach to charting our blueprint for life success.

For example, to neglect the giving, service, or social components of the life balance chart could easily result in self-absorption, and therefore, intra- and inter-personal stagnancy.

Unless a grain of wheat falls unto the earth it remains by itself alone.
-Jesus Christ

Similarly, to spend all of our time giving and serving, while neglecting our financial, personal health, and recreational needs is a recipe for disaster as well.

All work and no play makes Jack a dull boy,
All play and no work makes Jack a mere toy.
-Maria Edgeworth

Essentially, when seeking to blueprint well, we must remember to prioritize our lives in such a way that we keep first things first, while also remembering to include all of the important areas that promote personal well-being.

Keeping Our Priorities Straight

I still recall an informal meeting with my former sales director in which he pleaded with me to take a position out of state to help support company efforts to expand their presence there. The job would have meant a doubling of my income, but also required that I spend more time out of state than at home. I declined the position, not wishing to spend so much time away from my daughter. She was three years old at the time.

And since it was an informal meeting, I just happened to be holding my daughter on my lap. He was clearly upset about my decision and said (pointing to my daughter), "She is your problem, and the reason you will never make the kind of money you can potentially make, and to which you aspire." I looked at him and said, "She is not my problem, but rather, she is my daughter, and the most important reason for living!" I then challenged him that I would make even more money (working elsewhere!) all the while maintaining a significant day-to-day presence in my daughter's life.

Success Comes in Many Packages

We often equate success with financial wealth. Perhaps that is due to Western cultural values conditioning, combined with a common sense recognition that money is a means by which we can obtain so many of the things that we both need and want.

Money isn't the most important thing in life, but it's reasonably close to oxygen on the 'gotta have it' scale.

-Zig Ziglar

I don't mind admitting that I desire financial prosperity. Not so much for the money (as an end in itself), but rather, as a byproduct of having achieved the goal of becoming my best personal, professional, social, and spiritual self, as well as to provide a rewarding lifestyle for both my children and myself.

A few years ago, as I began blueprinting my reimmersion into the field of therapy, coaching, speaking, and writing, I realized there were several career options available to me—options that likely would have produced a higher income more quickly. However, the determining factor for me was that my work in this field would require every ounce of personal and professional development that I could muster; providing a catalyst towards growing into the kind of person, and making the sort of life contribution that I most desire in my heart of hearts. I can assure you, it wasn't the easiest route, but certainly the most gratifying in the long run.

Timeless Principles

This session, Blueprinting Well, together with this entire book, contains timeless principles that are transferable to virtually everyone, regardless of a person's sociocultural, economic, political, or religious background. And though definitions of what it means to be "a success" often vary from person to person, e.g., spiritual attainment; establishing meaningful and enduring relationships; outstanding service to humanity; or professional, social, and financial status, etc., we can all agree that in order to achieve success in any endeavor, total dedication and personal sacrifice must serve as prerequisites.

An Uncommon Definition of Success

For instance, the apostle Paul defined success as emanating from total dedication to the cross of Christ, and therefore, from the spiritual realm. He writes,

"For though I am free from all men, I have made myself a slave to all, that I might win the more . . . Do you not know that those who run in a race all run, but only one receives the prize? Run in such a way that you may win. And everyone who competes in the games exercises self control in all things. They do it to receive a perishable wreath, but we an imperishable. . . . Therefore I run in such a way, as not without aim; I box in such a way, as not beating the air; but I buffet my body and make it my slave, lest possibly, after I have preached to others, I myself should be disqualified. . . . I press on toward the goal for the prize of the upward call in Christ Jesus"

(1 Corinthians 9: 19, 23-27 and Philippians 3:14 respectively).

For Paul, the words of the Lord Jesus Christ, "For what will a man be profited, if he gains the whole world, and forfeits his soul? Or what will a man give in exchange for his soul?" served an ever present reminder of where his focus and priorities should rest.

From Homeless to Harvard

For Liz Murray, success meant breaking her family cycle of drug addiction, neglect, and homelessness.

After years of neglect, wherein Liz and her sister were exposed to their parents' drug abuse, and even having to resort to eating such a thing as toothpaste in order to fend off the pangs of hunger, she left home. Liz spent her adolescence in New York sleeping on the streets, in trains, and on the couches of friends. According to her, this was a frightening experience, despite the fact that homelessness coursed through her blood by virtue of her family's DNA. As an adolescent, her mother had also been homeless, and became addicted to drugs at an early age.

Liz recalled that her mother use to often tell her, "One day everything will get better for us. You will see." It was always "One day." But that day never came. In fact, matters grew worse before getting better.

At the age of sixteen Liz was served an unnerving wake-up call. In a September 9, 2010 interview aired on NPR's Talk of the Nation with host Jennifer Ludden, Liz recounted that after just having buried her mom, she was confronted with the increasingly obvious symmetry of both their lives paths. Liz, as one homeless and set adrift, stated, "I was re-living her life. I was re-creating a cycle that I knew had to change. I needed to break this cycle!"

Instead of allowing her painful life circumstances to thrust her further into hopelessness and despair—excusing herself as the product of defective genes, a victim of circumstance who could never possibly amount to anything—she chose to take control of her thoughts and life.

At that moment Liz made a life-transforming decision to get off the streets, return to school, and graduate with her high school diploma. In time, and with a lot of hard work and perseverance, she not only graduated from high school, but won a scholarship to Harvard. She graduated from there in 2009. Liz successfully broke the cycle of addiction, neglect, and homelessness that had destroyed her family.

I firmly believe that any man's finest hour—this greatest fulfillment to all he holds dear—is that moment when he has worked his heart out in a good cause and lies exhausted on the field of battle— victorious.

-Vince Lombardi

In her memoir *Breaking Night: A Memoir of Forgiveness, Survival, and My Journey from Homeless to Harvard*, Liz recounts her story in a moving and inspiring way.

Liz is now a motivational speaker and the founder of Manifest Living, an organization dedicated to inspiring hope and change in peoples' lives. She points out, "People often believe that their circumstances define who they are, when in reality, that is not the case. . . . People have so much more say-so, so much more control over their lives than they often realize."

Getting up is a choice!

With regards to your life, it is my hope that the Get Up! New Mind Synergy Formula for Success will prove helpful to this END.

AFTERWORD

Regardless of your present situation, there is hope for you. By applying the cognitive strategies so effective for transforming the forest of your mind, you can establish a healthy new thought life. Then, by creating a goals-centered life success blueprint, you can get back on track, and become more confident and successful than ever before. The new mind synergy formula for success has worked for numerous others, and it can work for you too.

Chances are you have already come to see your fallings and failures, as well as the pain and difficulties of life in a whole new and more hopeful light. Perhaps you have even discovered that it is perfectly okay to be you, and to embrace your life's journey as one of a kind. With such a mindset you can build on your strengths and successes, as well as your failures, and begin realizing your dreams for a brighter future.

Like so many others, as you begin working the steps that you've laid-out in your personal goals life success blueprint, your life will begin to virtually "take-off" in a positive new direction. Your friends and family will stand amazed as they witness this incredible transformation taking place.

Remember to associate with "eagles" in working towards your vision. Guard yourself from the negative people, places, and things that are often so sabotaging of your success. Consider obtaining a private coach, or join a group coaching program. There are strength and wisdom in numbers.

Also, bear in mind that a successful utilization of this formula means taking action. You must apply the exercises and techniques if you wish to succeed.

Keep your goals blueprint for life success and personal virtues development list well organized, and refer to them every single day. Make updates as needed.

The virtues of a positive attitude, courage, self-discipline, and persistence will strengthen you along the way.

Write this book's inspirational quotes in places where you are likely to see them often, and post images from magazines of people, places, things, and experiences that will enhance your vision for success.

Finally, remember to blueprint well.

Then . . . get moving!

Success,

-Dr. Miller

ACKNOWLEDGMENTS

I owe many thanks to Joyce Maltais, Ph.D., for her leadership role in editing and proofreading the initial phases of the manuscript. Phyllis Eckhardt was instrumental in proofreading at a time when I desperately needed a fresh set of eyes!

Dr. Paul Larsen and Mr. Ken Savage were both a tremendous encouragement, especially during the initial stages of the books development—our discussions helped clarify the reality that it is impossible to become fully spiritual, without first becoming fully human, and vice versa.

Thank you to Dr. Christine Tanimura of California Southern University for your confidence in me and your encouragement along the way. You take the role of Academic Advisor to a whole new level!

Also, thanks to my clients. Without you this book would not have been possible. You are all so brave, so committed, and such a joy to work with—keep growing!

Finally, thank you to the staff at WestBow Press for making this book possible.

VISIT DR. MILLER ONLINE:

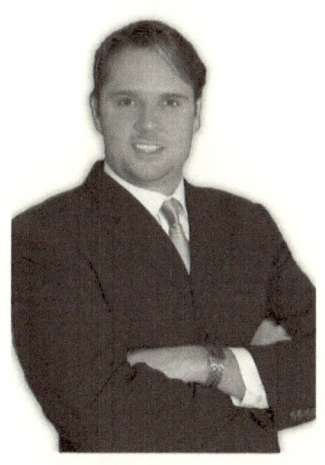

www.coachingwithchris.net

*Sign-up for a FREE subscription to his monthly newsletter.

References

Preface

1. Amen, D. (2002). *Healing the hardware of the soul* (pp. 5-7, 18). New York, NY: Free Press.

2. Boyle, M. (2010). November 28. *Cognitive enhancers*. www.cogsci. ucsd.edu.

3. Cacioppo, J., Bernston, G., Sheridan, J., & McClintock, M. (2001). Multilevel analyses of human behavior: Social neuroscience and the complementing nature of social and biological approaches. In J. Cacioppo (Ed.), *Foundations in social neuro-science* (pp. 21-46). Cambridge, M.A: MIT Press.

4. Foster, P.L., & Cairns, J. (1994, November) The occurrence of heritable Mu excisions in starving cells of *Escherichia coli*. *The EMBO Journal, 13* (21), 5240-5244.

5. Hill, N. (1937). *Think & grow rich*. The Ralston Society.

6. Jensen, E. (2005). *Teaching with the brain in mind* (p. 11). Alexandria, VA: ASCD.

7. Reik, W., Dean, W., & Walter, J. (2001). Epigenetic reprogramming in mammalian development. *Science*, 293, 1089-1093.

8. Suomi, S. (1999). Attachment in rhesus monkeys. In J. Cassidy & P. Shaver (Eds.), *Handbook of attachment* (pp. 181-197). New York: Guilford Press.

9. Wikipedia.com, Ergonomics.com, & Word IQ.com. *Hybrid definition of synergy.*

Introduction n/a

Session 1

1. Feuerstein, R., Rand, Y., Feuerstein, R.S., *You love me!!...don't accept me as I am: Helping the low functioning person excel.* Jerusalem, Israel: ICELP & the Company for the enhancement of Mediated Learning Ltd.

2. Jensen, E. (2005). *Teaching with the brain in mind* (pp. 11, 75). Alexandria, VA: ASCD.

3. Kubler-Ross, E. (1969). *On death and dying.* New York, NY: Scribner.

4. Leaf, C. (2009). *The gift in you* (pp. 11-12). Southlake, TX: Inprov, LTd.

5. Miller, C. (1999) *Foundations Four (4) Family Success.* Riverside, CA.: LWM.

6. Tracy, B. (2003) *The ultimate goals program.* Niles, IL: Nightingale-Conant.

Session 2

1. Burns, D. (1993). *Ten days to self-esteem.* New York, NY: Harper Collins.

2. Data Accountability Center (http://www.ideadata.org/PartBChild Count.asp) 23 June 2010.

3. Howard, P. (2000). *The owner's manual for the brain* (pp. 351-352, 790). Marietta, GA: Bard Press.

4. Jensen, E. (2005). *Teaching with the brain in mind.* (pp. 75). Alexandria, VA.: ASCD.

5. Kimura, D. and Hampson, E. (1990, April). *Neural and hormonal mechanisms mediating sex differences in cognition.* Research Bulletin No. 689. London, Ontario, Canada; Department of Psychology, University of Western Ontario.

6. Kolata, G.B. (1976). "Brain Biochemistry: Effects of diet." *Science,* 192, 41-42. 6. Leaf, C. (2009). *The gift in you* (pp. 11, 12, 31, 162). Southlake, TX.: Inprov, LTd.

7. National Institute for Learning Development (NILD).

8. Smalley, G., Smalley, G., Cretsinger, D., and Cretsinger, M (2010). *The heart of remarriage.* Wheaton, IL.: Publishers, INC.

9. Thompson, J.G. (1988). *The psychology of emotions.* New York: Plenum

10. Tracy, B. (2003). *The ultimate goals program.* Niles, IL: Nightingale-Conant.

11. U.S. Department of Education, 25th annual report to Congress.

Session 3

1. Eriksson, P.S., Perfilieva, E., Bjork-Ericksson, T. et al. 1998. Neurogenesis in the adult human hippocampus. *Nature Medicine, 4,* pp. 1313-1317.

2. Gould, E., Beylin, A., Tanapat, P., Reeves, A., & Shors, T.J. 1999. Learning enhances adult neurogenesis in the hippocampal formation. *Nature neuroscience, 2,* pp. 260-265.

3. Hardy, S., Seeds of success magazine. *The greatest goal and purpose in life.* (2010, September 7).

4. Holiday, R. (1990). *Mechanisms for the control of gene activity during development.* Biol. Rev. Cambr. Philos. Soc. 65, 431-471.

5. Jaguar Educational (2010).

6. Jensen, E. (2005). *Teaching with the brain in mind.* Alexandria, VA: ASCD.

7. Kempermann, G., & Gage, F.H. 1999. New nerve cells for the adult brain. *Scientific American, 280,* pp. 48-53.

8. Restak, R.M., (1994). *The modular brain.* York, NY: Macmillan.

9. Schwartz, J.M. & Begley, S. (2002). *The mind & the brain: neuroplasticity and the power of mental force* (pp. 8, 111). New York, NY: HarperCollins.

Session 4

1. Diamond, M., & Hopson, J. (1995). *How to . . . Magic trees of the mind.* Penguin, USA.

2. Leaf, C. (2009). *The gift in you* (pp. 143-147). Southlake, TX: Inprov, LTd.

3. Leaf Interview with Ali Brown *Clean out your brain! control your toxic thoughts and emotions for best success.* (July 13, 2010).

4. Nader, K., Schafe, G.E. et al. (2000). "Fear memories require protein synthesis in the amygdala for reconsolidation after retrieval." *Nature* 406, 722-726.

5. Tonson & Taylor (2007). "Molecular mechanisms of memory consolidation." *Nature Reviews Neuorscience,* 8, 262-275.

Session 5

1. Amen, D. (2002). *Healing the hardware of the soul* (p. 148, 150-155). New York, NY. Free Press.

2. Tracy, B. (2003). *The ultimate goals program.* Niles, IL: Nightingale-Conant.

Session 6 n/a

Session 7

1. Hill, N. (1937). *Think and grow rich.* Ralston Publishing Society.

2. Mark H. MacCormack. *What they don't teach you at Harvard business school.*

3. Marden, O.S. (1894) *Pushing to the front.*

4. Shultz, Dayan, & Montague (2002). From Jensen p. 77.

5. Tracy, B. (2003). *The ultimate goals program.* Niles, IL: Nightingale-Conant.

Session 8

1. Heim, P., & Murphy, S. (2001). *In the company of women: Turning workplace conflict into powerful alliances.* New York, NY: Penguin Putnam Inc.

2. Insight Publishing/Interviews Conducted by David E. Wright (2004). *Conversations on success* (pp. 136).

3. Tracy, B. (2003). *The ultimate goals program.* Niles, IL: Nightingale-Conant.

Session 9

1. Hill, N. (1937). *Think and grow rich.* Ralston Publishing Society.

2. Tracy, B. (2003). *The ultimate goals program.* Niles, IL: Nightingale-Conant.

Session 10

1. Amen, D. (2002). *Healing the hardware of the soul* (p. 150-155). New York, NY. Free Press.

Session 11

1. NPR Interview with former Secretary Of State Condoleezza Rice.

2. Today Show Interview Online.

Session 12

1. Miller, R. (2005) Moral courage: definition and development. *Ethics Resource Center.* www.ethics.org.

2. Poor Richard's Almanack (1732).

3. Beckwith, J., & Koukl, G. (1998). *Relativism: feet firmly planted in mid-air.* Baker.

Session 13

1. Mischell, Walter. Stanford Marshmallow Study.

Session 14

1. Marden, O.S. (1894). *Pushing to the front.*

2. Taylor, S.E. (1991, July). Asymmetrical effects of positive and negative events: The mobilization-minimization hypothesis. *Pyshcological Bullettin, 110*(1), 67-85.

Session 15 Conclusion

1. NPR interview with Liz Murray, September 09, 2010.

www.ingramcontent.com/pod-product-compliance
Lightning Source LLC
Chambersburg PA
CBHW030318290526
45785CB00001B/419